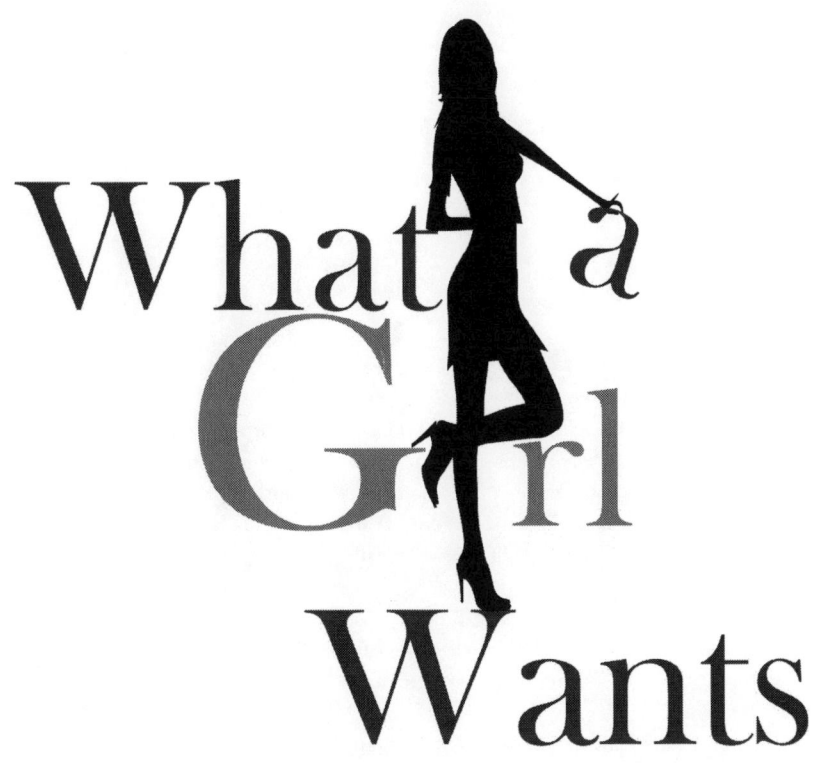

What a Girl Wants

The Good Girl's Guide to *Great* Sex

SARA BOLDEN, DPT, WCS

Copyright © 2014 Sara Bolden.

All rights reserved. No part of this book may be reproduced, stored, or transmitted by any means—whether auditory, graphic, mechanical, or electronic—without written permission of both publisher and author, except in the case of brief excerpts used in critical articles and reviews. Unauthorized reproduction of any part of this work is illegal and is punishable by law.

ISBN: 978-1-3045-8748-0 (sc)
ISBN: 978-1-4834-0602-2 (e)

Because of the dynamic nature of the Internet, any web addresses or links contained in this book may have changed since publication and may no longer be valid. The views expressed in this work are solely those of the author and do not necessarily reflect the views of the publisher, and the publisher hereby disclaims any responsibility for them.

Any people depicted in stock imagery provided by Thinkstock are models, and such images are being used for illustrative purposes only.
Certain stock imagery © Thinkstock.

Lulu Publishing Services rev. date: 01/23/2014

CONTENTS

Acknowledgements vii

Introduction
THE GOOD GIRLS' GUIDE TO GREAT SEX ix

Chapter One
WHAT'S UP WITH "DOWN THERE"? 1

Chapter Two
THE BRAIN: THE BIGGEST SEX ORGAN IN THE FEMALE BODY 9

Chapter Three
LOCATION, LOCATION, LOCATION! 19

Chapter Four
HANDLE WITH CARE…AND YOUR VAGINA WILL THANK
YOU FOR IT! 25

Chapter 5
THE BIG "O": WHY CAN'T I HAVE ONE? 31

Chapter Six
WHAT'S GOING ON DOWN THERE? WHEN THINGS ARE
JUST NOT FEELING RIGHT 41

Chapter Seven
WHAT ARE MY OPTIONS? TREATMENT AND
MANAGEMENT FOR PAINFUL INTERCOURSE 51
    PART 1: TREATMENT CHOICES
    PART 2: STAYING CONNECTED WITH INTIMACY

Chapter Eight
I LIKE IT LIKE THAT! ORTHOPEDIC CONSIDERATIONS FOR
INTIMACY 61

Chapter Nine
DEAD IN THE BED? GET YOUR GROOVE BACK! 69

Chapter Ten
STRIVING FOR BETTER 77

Chapter Eleven
FAQ'S: REAL QUESTIONS FROM REAL WOMEN 81

References 89

ACKNOWLEDGEMENTS

There are many individuals that I'd like to acknowledge and extend my appreciation to for supporting and encouraging me throughout this process. The first being my inspiration for even writing this book! That would be my heavenly father, God. Had He not placed the idea in my heart and encouraged me through multiple people and avenues, many times over, to write this book, it probably would not have happened. I am who I am and I do what I do all because of Him! All glory and honor be to God!

I would like to thank my best friend and love of my life for always supporting, inspiring and motivating me. Kelvin, I love doing life with you! You are such a wonderful man, husband and father. I count each day with you a blessing! Thank you for being here for me and encouraging me when I wanted to throw in the towel!

Mary and Joe Graziano, you are the best mom and dad a girl could ever have! I'm sure you never dreamed that your daughter would grow up one day to write a book on how to have great sex, but it didn't seem to deter your support! You have always been a source of strength and guidance that has kept me grounded my entire life. Thank you for decades of encouragement and unconditional love!

To my mentors and colleagues, Cora Huitt and Karen Abraham, you are the reason I love this profession! You both have brilliant minds and kind, compassionate spirits. You inspire me to be the best I can be and help me maximize my potential! I am sincerely grateful to both of you for nurturing me throughout my professional career and during this book writing process.

There are others that have been instrumental in dropping seeds of encouragement and wisdom along the way. Those "others" include my friends and family, patients and staff from Women First Rehabilitation and colleagues from various healthcare specialties. You have prayed for me, advised me, comforted me and cheered me on! I am truly blessed to know you and have you in my corner. Thank you! Thank you! Thank you!

INTRODUCTION

The Good Girls' Guide to Great Sex

Sex is like coffee. The first few cups are often fresh and invigorating. You're left feeling energized and ready to conquer the world. You suddenly feel more efficient and confident to finish the tasks of your day. However, as time passes, its potency and lasting effects diminish and you're often left desiring more from your coffee than ever before. And sometimes, it becomes stale and ineffective leaving a bitter aftertaste. You suddenly wake up one day thinking, "We're not at Starbucks anymore, Dorothy." The kind of sex you had when you first encountered your true love is no longer exciting, fresh or rejuvenating. Although you love your mate, you find yourself having sex because you're "supposed to" or "ought to". Overtime, you start finding "legitimate" reasons to avoid it….headache, exhaustion, the children, your-mother-in-law-is-sleeping-down-the-hall, etc. It can become unfulfilling, even disappointing…leaving a bitter aftertaste.

Just like adding a flavor shot to coffee, sex can be brought back to life. It can be resurrected to become the most exhilarating and fulfilling aspect of your marriage. Even if you've been married for decades, there is hope for new discoveries and sensations you've never experienced…or at least not in the past 10-15 years. And get this…are you sitting down…after learning about how to get your groove back, YOU may even be the one initiating intercourse. I know, very alarming, but that is the goal of this book.

What a Girl Wants was written with women in mind. Women like you. Women like me. Our bodies were purposed for sexual intercourse with specific anatomy that was divinely designed for the sole intention of producing sexual pleasure. That means, you were made to have sex, and not just sex, but GOOD sex; the kind of sex that makes you feel incredible, leaving you desiring more. It's the kind of intimacy that has you smiling at work, giggling in the grocery store, and daydreaming about the next encounter. Yeah, you remember those days, it's making you smile right now.

The key to unlocking a world of heightened pleasures and marital "bliss" is sitting right in your lap. You've had it all along. You were even born with it! It defines your sexuality and is the symbol of femininity. We're talking about your pelvis which includes your sexual genitalia as well as your pelvic floor muscles, surrounding tissues, glands, nerves, blood supply and hormones. It is the heart of your womanhood, yet the least understood by most women. If we don't know how our own bodies work, we certainly can't rely on men to figure it out.

Who teaches men to have sex anyway? Their friends? Brothers? Uncles? And who taught those guys? Their friends? Their brothers? Their uncles? The point is, most men have no clue about a woman's body. Can we blame them? They don't have a vagina. From their first encounter, their challenge is figuring out how to adequately pleasure their lady all the while trying to appear like they've known how to do it all along. A lot of times it comes down to trial and error. There's nothing wrong with that, but it can often lead to frustration for both parties involved.

Most individuals, both men and women, have some idea of what sex *is* prior to actually becoming sexually active. These "ideas" typically stem from what's portrayed by Hollywood, on TV shows and/or in the pornography industry. What's wrong with that, you ask? Well, let's start with the obvious. It's acting... not real. Second, it's often created and produced by men for men. These sexual media outlets are geared primarily towards men with few, if any, images of real, deep emotional connections, trust or commitment between characters. You know, the stuff women really find sexy. Sex is portrayed as spontaneous, non-committal, acts of intense thrusts ending in climatic release for both parties involved. Truth be told, this is rarely the case for the average, committed couple. And guess what, we women want more than that.

Wanting more and knowing how to get more has been a problem for women since the beginning of time. In fact, it's such a big problem that most women stop searching for better and end up settling for less than gratifying. What many women don't know is that sex plays a big role in her overall health and life span. Surprising, but true! Countless studies show that sexual intercourse can improve blood pressure, increase circulation, boost the immune system, decrease depression and anxiety and even improve your cholesterol. Not only that, but you can burn up to 214 calories every time you do the hanky panky! *Shut-UP!*

In a study that looked at the relationship between sex and death, researchers followed approximately 1000 men over a 10 year span and found that the more orgasms they had the longer they lived. However, for women, complementary studies showed that it wasn't the **quantity**, or how often women had sex, that increased their life's longevity, rather the **quality** of sex that does the trick.

If women enjoyed sex, then they lived longer, happier lives…by up to 50%! *And you thought it was a waste of time.* Finding out how to enjoy sex is not only fun and refreshing but adds years to your life, too! Now, there's a reason to pursue a better sex life!

What a Girl Wants is just the guide women have been looking for. This book is intended to inform, enlighten, confirm and inspire women regardless of age, marital longevity, education or social status. It will help answer questions about your body, educate you on the pelvic floor, sexual health and motivate you to reconnect with your mate on new intimate levels. If you're not having really good intercourse or you just need a "love boost", keep reading. You will NOT be disappointed. By the end of this book, you will have a fresh, up-to-date understanding of your body and learn to coach your partner with direction and purpose. The time is now! No more pretending to be asleep! Let this be a new beginning to your happily ever after!

CHAPTER ONE

What's up with "Down There"?

Bill glances over at his lovely wife from across the dining room table with a look of complete satisfaction. Once again, she has surpassed his expectations with another delicious mid-week dinner. It's been a while since the two of them have shared a meal alone without competing for attention with the kids, out-of-town visitors or unannounced neighbors. Bill reaches for her hand and gives it a gentle squeeze followed by "the eye"; you know which one….the "you-look-better-than-the-steak-I-just-ate" eye. She meets his goofy smile with her own version of "the eye", the "are-you-kidding-me?-I-just-finished-a-long-day-at-work-only-to-come-home-and-slave-over-the-stove,-not-to-mention-I'll-be-staying-up-late-to-clean-the-kitchen" eye. Although, she loves her husband, she does not desire sexual intimacy, because more times than not, it provides little to no pleasure for her and, quite frankly, she's exhausted. She wonders to herself, "Is there something wrong with me? I feel dead down there."

VaJay-Jay, Hoo-Ha, Coozie, Twinkie, Flower, Tutu, Cooter or whatever nickname you have given your female parts, you must first know what's "down there," before you can truly find, appreciate and experience your pleasure zones. Knowing these little intricate details of your body is half the battle! The other half is figuring out the right combinations that adequately stimulate and arouse you. Having a tool like this book and understanding the love connection between your body and sexual intimacy can also serve as the perfect dialogue opener between you and your mate. When you both are on the same page, there's bursting potential for a whole new world of exploration and excitement.

Let's start by identifying the pelvis, vulva and the pelvic floor. You might be asking yourself, "I have a floor?" and the answer is a resounding "YES!" Your pelvic floor plays a critical role in sexual intimacy. It is made up of power-generating muscles that function three-fold: 1) to support your organs, 2) open/close your urethra and rectum and 3) aids in producing the most euphoric of all sexual sensations, the orgasm. During an orgasm, these pelvic floor muscles can produce few or many repetitive, quick contractions. In most cases, the stronger these muscles are and the more endurance they have to activity, the more intense your orgasm can be and the increased likelihood there is of having multiple orgasms. Who wouldn't want that!?!? However, we must not stop our investigation here! These pelvic floor muscles do not work in solo to do such a thing. No, these muscles are only a portion of the bigger picture. For each woman, it is the unique, and individualized, combination of stimulating the correct anatomical structures and establishing your frame of mind that helps take you to heightened pleasures. In essence, during intercourse, the pelvis, vulva, pelvic floor muscles and the brain work in symphony to produce an ultimate goal of intense sexual pleasure and, often, orgasm.

Let's break these components down further to see how we can improve their sexual potential. In the most simplistic terms, your pelvis, or also known as the pelvic girdle, consisting of two hip bones, called innominates, connected in the front by the pubic symphysis and in the back by your sacrum and coccyx (the "tailbone"). These two innominates (a.k.a. hip bones) are then held together by ligaments, pelvic floor muscles and their corresponding tendons and connective tissues. Its job is to provide a solid, supportive structure that allows us to tolerate weight bearing activities such as walking, standing, sitting, kneeling, side-lying, etc. As you can imagine, the pelvic girdle plays an important role in the kind of sexual positions you can tolerate during intercourse. If you've been having sex in the same position for years because "that's just the way we've done it," then it may be time to discover new positions.

Unfortunately, your 20-something year old hips are not the same as your 40-something year old hips, especially if they've played a role in carrying and birthing a child (or children). More often than not, things have "shifted" a little (or A LOT) over the years and the sexual positions you once adored in the past may, today, be increasing your back or tailbone pain. Not only does the pelvic girdle provide a good platform for trying various intimate positions, it also serves as home-base for the more obvious pleasure zones, like the clitoris.

Ah, the clitoris, the most talked about erogenous spot on a woman's body. It is here that most men believe is the key to taking his woman swiftly to her climatic sanctuary. And, often, it is! However, the clitoris is not the kind of zone that can be aggressively pursued, at least not initially. With six to eight thousand nerve endings all bundled up in a teeny, tiny nodule, a little "courtship" is necessary rather than a full, all-out, frontal engagement. Utilizing the entire vulva area with gentle and frequent "visitations" to the clitoris will ultimately create the best sustainable arousal and complete satisfaction.

As you can see here in the bottom image of Figure 1, the clitoris is much bigger than what is visible to the eye.

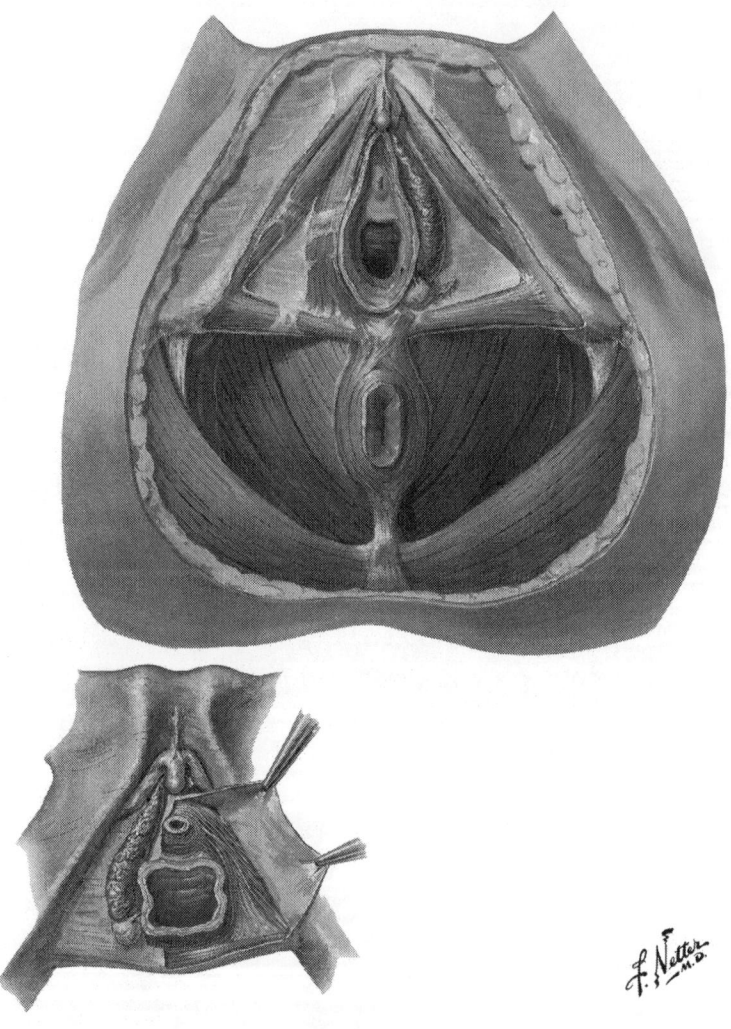

Figure 1

It extends into the vagina and separates away from its apex into two tail-like structures called crura. It has contractile tissue and is affluent in blood supply (which, by the way, makes for a lovely set-up to produce an orgasm). Upon arousal, the clitoris becomes saturated with oxygen-rich blood flow which further awakens neighboring nerve endings. Its' delicate, visible structure is protected by a fleshy hood which is retracted as it becomes engorged with blood and reaches its fully erected state. (Yes, Ladies, we can have erections, too). The superficial pelvic floor muscles are attached here and assist in making the clitoris erect as well as aid in the production of an orgasm.

As mentioned before, the majority of men are, at minimal, aware of the location of the clitoris….you can't miss it, really. However, most are unfamiliar with the sexual response and full arousing potential found in her neighboring counter-parts. We call this visible genital area, the vulva. The vulva is the external genital that you can see if you were to examine yourself with a hand held mirror (See Figure 2). It is here that you will find the inner and outer folds of the vagina (i.e. labia minora and majora, respectively), the clitoris, urethra and the vaginal opening.

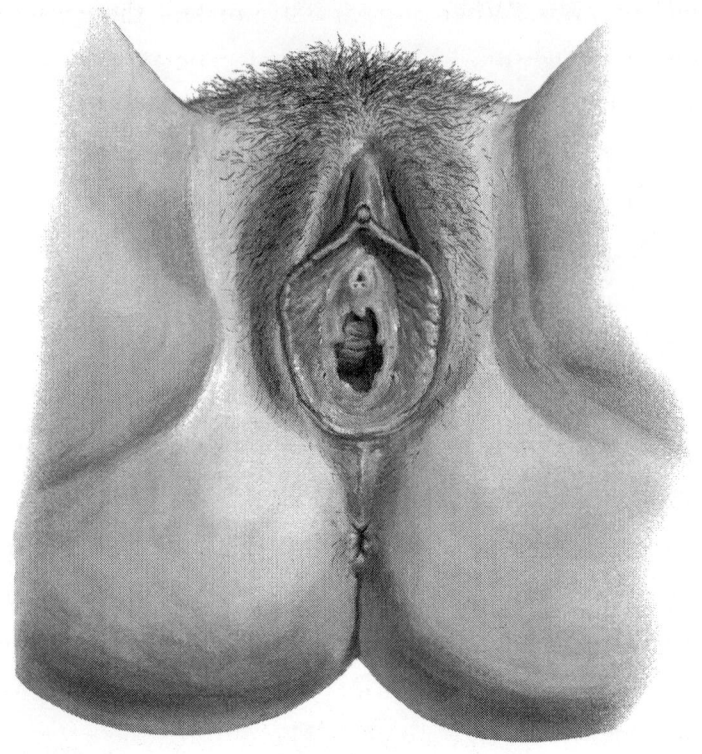

Figure 2

What you can't see, but is of equal importance, is a delicate lattice work of blood and nerve supply woven throughout the pelvis, as well as the lubricating vestibular glands. In fact, the vulva is where we find structures, dense with nerve endings, which have no other purpose than for sexual stimulation, such as with the clitoris. These areas are so densely filled with innervation, that they have the ability to produce the most incredible pleasure or intense, excruciating pain. That is why it is necessary to approach the vagina with careful precaution and delicate caress. Other areas infiltrated with nerve endings include the inner folds (labia minor), the area where the crura of the clitoris begin to merge together and the anus. When properly stimulated, these nerve endings trigger a cascade of events that increase blood flow, trigger internal vaginal lubrication and prepare the vaginal opening for entry.

During arousal, changes in the vulva can be observed right before your very eyes. There is a rush of blood to the area, which will change the color of tissue to a deep pink or crimson (depending on a woman's overall skin tone). The vulva becomes moistened with vaginal lubrication and the labia majora becomes puffy and extended outward unveiling the vaginal opening. The pelvic floor will begin to produce small muscle contractions. In some women, this process takes seconds to minutes whereas for others, um…well, let's just say patience is a virtue. No matter what category you are thinking of placing yourself, please note that every woman is different and each encounter may produce different results, even if it's with the same mate! "Why is that?" you might be asking yourself. The largest sex organ in the female body is the brain.

CHAPTER TWO

The Brain: The Biggest Sex Organ in the Female Body

For women, there are two main aspects of sexual pleasure, the physical and the mental. Let me preface the next few paragraphs by setting a few things straight. First, for females, sexual touch is not created equal. What stimulates and pleasures one woman does not always produce the same response in another. Why? Perception is the culprit. You must *perceive* the tissues being stimulated as arousing and safe, at minimal, before you can respond in a pleasurable way. If you do not perceive these tissues as erotic or sensual, maybe due to an injury or past sexual trauma, then these areas will provide little to downright unfavorable pleasurable sensations. The injury and/or traumatic event must be dealt with and healed, thus changing your perception of that particular body region, prior to utilizing these sensitive areas during intimacy. If you believe your injury to be more musculoskeletal related, then a women's health physical therapist may be the perfect solution to getting you back into action. If you are struggling to get beyond the mental and emotional trauma of your injury, then a sex therapist (i.e. a psychologist, physician or licensed counselor with specialized training in sex and relationships) is probably the most appropriate referral. The best recovery observed for someone who has encountered a physical and emotional injury to the pelvis is one being treated through a multidisciplinary approach (gynecologist, women's health physical therapist, and sex therapist, at minimal). Until these areas are healed, you may always struggle with sexual intimacy.

Nonetheless, even without physical and/or emotional complications, each woman's body responds differently to various stimulants. What feels sensual and exciting to one woman may feel boring, irritating or painful to another. This sometimes happens even within your own body at any given time. Get this, sometimes the touching and kissing that had your heart pounding and toes tingling on day one, can barely keep you awake the following day. WHY? Because mood, libido, alertness and sensuality begin in your brain!

The brain is the motherboard to which everything derives. It is a very complex system that continues, at times, to baffle medical researchers in its abilities. Since perceptions are individualized to every person, it is easy to see how each woman may experience sexuality uniquely. Additionally, women will experience different responses to sexual stimuli at different times of the month based on normal, cyclic hormonal changes as well as hormonal changes due to menopause, day to day stresses, and/or environmental situations. Oh, and let's not discount the effects of perceived self-image. Having a bad hair day? Did your face decide to break out unexpectedly? Feeling stuffed in your "fat" jeans? The way you feel about yourself can kill a libido without hesitation and with consistency like no other. These are common aspects of normal life that you should recognize and adjust or adapt to when choosing a time and day to be intimate. In other words, expect some days to have no sex, others to have good sex and some days to have incredible, "I-am-having-an out-of-body-experience" sex!

I know what you might be thinking, "Oh, great…If my brain is responsible for determining whether or not I get to have great sex, I'm hopeless." After all, you can't change your brain, right? Well, the answer is yes and no. You can NOT, or shall I say SHOULD not, try to change your brain's physical properties (that would be bad…very, very, bad….not to mention life threatening). However, you CAN (and SHOULD) try to change some of the chemical properties, temporarily, as it pertains to arousal and sexual intimacy; and thus, help change your "perception", if you will. Let us not undermine the fact that there may be major hormonal imbalances contributing to this lack of sexual interest, i.e. low estrogen and/or testosterone levels are two of the biggest culprits. Low hormonal production and/or hormonal imbalances are common problems of aging, but should not be accepted as "normal". Although pharmaceutical management of hormonal imbalances is an option and may be necessary for some, there are many non-pharmaceutical remedies that women can do to increase her libido.

Let's first address your overall impression of sex. If you come into the bed with the idea that it's going to be boring, lifeless and uneventful, then it probably will be. It's a concept called confirmation bias. Confirmation bias is a tendency of an individual to gather information that confirms a preset bias in his or her mind. So, in other words, if you feel that sex is always boring, then you will look for ways to confirm that sex is boring. You may even create or rehearse those findings in your mind as they are happening in real time. For example, you may say to yourself,

"Here we go again." "He's going to do the same stuff he always does. I'm going to pretend like I'm enjoying it so he can hurry up." "See, he never changes it up." Perhaps he never changes it up because you are pretending to enjoy it. Therefore, he thinks he's doing a good job. See how this could get dangerous? If sex has been unsatisfying for a long time, it's very easy to slip into confirmation bias mode. It is your responsibility to communicate to your mate about your likes/dislikes so he has the opportunity to change his behavior. Also, try changing your bias thinking into something more positive and rehearse those thoughts while making love. This helps to set the stage for your brain's chemistry and creates an environment to maximize the release of all the love hormones released during intimacy. Confirm, in your brain, all the sexy acts that are unfolding on your body as they happen. You might say to yourself, "I love it when he kisses me here." "It feels so good when he touches me there," or "I love the way his body feels against mine." etc.

There are several things that you can do with and without your partner to momentarily change the chemistry of your brain. Certain sex neurotransmitters and hormones, such as oxytocin and dopamine, are released in the brain when you engage in certain activities such as massage, hugging/kissing, relaxation techniques, meditation, dancing/exercising or fantasizing about your next love encounter. Men are really quite good at this fantasizing part! It doesn't take much for men to have their brains baptized in neurohormones with preparedness of sex, which physically manifests below the belt, in a matter of seconds. In fact, if they brush against in the couch the wrong way, they'll be on a manhunt to locate their unsuspecting wives to cop-a-feel....or more. In the September 2011 issue of *Psychology Today* magazine, statistics report that more than 50% of men think about having sex 5-7 times a day. However, most men would argue that those statistics are a little on the low side. *Go figure.*

Unfortunately, most women are not so good at this. At minimal, it takes quite a bit of intentional effort to get us going in the right direction mentally. We are so busy multitasking our lives and our children's lives and perhaps our close friends or co-worker's lives that we have forgotten the necessity of taking time to prepare our own minds and bodies for sexual intimacy. Most of us don't even know how or where to begin! The thought of having to do this kind of preparation is down-right overwhelming and time-consuming. Your libido, which once could be lit easily like a Fourth of July sparkler, now resembles a Crockpot turned to the "12 hours" setting. This might be okay, if we took the time to prepare ourselves for the full 12 hours. The problem is most of us are trying to operate and respond sexually after 10 minutes, or less, of Crock-potting! Don't fret, Ladies, once you know a few key "tricks" to increasing your arousal, the mental preparations will become much easier and more naturally for you.

Okay, so how do we do this? What are the tricks? First, do a little self-evaluating. Are you someone who likes fragrance, music, lighting, role-playing, massaging or taste-testing? Perhaps a little of this and/or a little of that? Then, first, prepare your mind for intimacy by tapping into your senses and knowing your desires. Before he even gets home from work, appeal to your senses in as many ways as possible. Stimulating one or more of your five senses will help facilitate relaxation, decrease stress and awaken your libido. Naturally, if you are someone who cannot tolerate fragrant candles or flowers, you should not incorporate the sense of smell into your preparedness. Likewise, if you remember the best sex you ever had with your soul mate to be the time you were on the beach during your honeymoon, then go get a sound machine with ocean waves! Buy candles and/or some simple props or lingerie to remind you of the sexy, steamy nights before children.

The next step in creating and enhancing your libido is letting go of some mental hang-ups about yourself and/or your partner. You probably don't look or feel the same as you did when you first started dating or when you got married, neither does your husband. While we, women, will beat ourselves up with the idea of returning our bodies (and faces) back to our teenage years, there is something you need to know. There have been many studies and polls asking men to describe the kind of woman that turns them on. In fact, hundreds of studies have investigated the type of female bodies men find most attractive and the results speak for themselves. An overwhelming majority, (one published study reports an astonishing 80%[3]), of men conclude that they prefer, and are more sexually aroused by, women who are curvy and/or voluptuous compared to skinny women. Ladies, if "voluptuous" is how you would describe yourself today, know you are still attractive and desired by most men in this country, more importantly, by YOUR man. Please do not misconstrue this as permission to become a couch potato eating Bon Bons. The importance of exercise is crucial on so many levels. It decreases the risks of heart disease, maintains and aids with weight loss, decreases risks of certain cancers, decreases depression and/or anxiety and, as you have just learned, increases the release of sex hormones which, in turn, increases your libido…not to mention it will also improve your ability to achieve an orgasm (*Can I get a hey, hey?*).

The third step in improving your libido and sexual sensations is to have the "more is better" mentality during foreplay. You remember what foreplay is, right? Right? *(Long awkward pause).* Well, foreplay is the cuddling, kissing, massaging, teasing, caressing, nibbling, dancing and the whispering of sweet nothings that you used to do when you were dating and first married. It's a necessary component of sexual intercourse.

During foreplay, and transitioning into intercourse, women will experience significant arousal if her erogenous zones are breached and heighten sexual pleasure if several erotic zones are stimulated at the same time. Stimulating multiple arousing zones (to include the breasts, clitoris, inner thighs, ear lobes, neck, abdomen, etc.) at the same time helps to release dopamine and oxytocin which are precursors and facilitators for intense sexual pleasure and orgasms. However, this could get tricky…depending on how many zones you are trying to stimulate at once. Unless you're married to an octopus, you may decide to have your mate stimulate one or two of your favorite arousing zones and/or help him out with a little self-stimulation. <*Gasp*> Self-stimulation!?!?!? Yes, I know, it's very taboo to discuss, but there are various methods of self-stimulation that can be utilized with your partner's participation and, of course, dependent on your comfort level.

Some women find it difficult, or uncomfortable, to look at or touch their own vaginas. The idea of self-stimulation has never been contemplated or explored. This may account for the lack of knowledge regarding which areas of the vulva and/or vagina are most exciting and stimulating to you. Before writing this concept off, know that self-stimulation can still involve your husband and can be instrumental in helping you achieve fantastic orgasms. It can be a very effective aspect of your foreplay and intercourse experience. It is an important key to discovering which parts of the vulva and vagina will respond best to his touch.

The kind of self-stimulation I will discuss, and encourage, is typically the most comfortable and accepted by women and is not performed solo. In fact, it's much better when your mate is involved. For you, it will serve as an effective way to discover what feels good, the amount of pressure that is needed to make you feel aroused and the type of stimulation that will get you to orgasm. For him, it's foreplay and education. Start by lying comfortably on your back. Use pillows to support your thighs and legs. Then, take your mate's well lubricated penis and gently explore your vulvar tissues. Explore up and down the entire vulva in a circular motion. When you get to that place that makes you blush, concentrate your circles in that spot. You may find that you prefer fast, small circles here or firm, vertical strokes. It doesn't matter what formula you use as long as you are feeling pleasure. Often, this kind of activity will produce enough pleasure and stimulation to cause an orgasm…and not just for you! The tip of the male penis is loaded with nerve endings, more than any other place on his genitalia. Often, when practicing this "self-stimulating" technique, both of you are able to reach climatic bliss and sexual delight!

When you experience this kind of sexual satisfaction and oneness with your spouse, it will have you excited and anticipating your next love encounter. Anticipation, alone, has the power to generate the entire arousal process….vaginal lubrication, increased blood flow, mild muscle contractions, fantasizing, etc. There are entire books describing how the magic of anticipation can improve your libido and enhance, even save, your marriage. So, if tonight's gonna be a "good" night, then start "crock-potting" early in your day. Leave your partner a love letter on the bathroom sink, send him a steamy email, buy yourself a sexy negligee, prepare the candles, listen to "your" song and turn down the lights.

Whether it be creating a sexy environment with incense and music, or meeting with your doctor to discuss if you are hormonally imbalanced, decide in your mind, to be intentional about improving your libido. It is not going to turn on by itself. It requires experimenting and consistency to discover the right recipe for arousal. Remember, the more you practice, the easier it gets. The easier it gets the more fun it is. Be creative, try something new, but whatever you do, don't give up.

CHAPTER THREE

Location, Location, Location!

Just like a cottage in acres of plush grasslands, luxurious cabins overlooking snow-peaked mountains or white, sandy, beachfront property, finding the perfect location to achieve your ultimate stimulation and sexual arousal is worth its weight in gold. Thankfully, women have several "hot spots" in and around the vagina that serve as exceptional venues for pleasure. There are two "spots" inside and two "spots" outside that have the potential of bringing ultimate arousal and heightened stimulation. However, not all women will respond to these places in the same way. My advice; if at first you don't succeed, try, try ANOTHER SPOT.

Most women, and men, have some knowledge of the whereabouts of the famous G-spot, but what they don't know is the majority of women do not like their G-spots stimulated <GASP>. If you are a woman reading this book you may be silently thinking to yourself, "No kidding, Sherlock." But the real question is why? The G-spot, a.k.a. Gräfenberg Spot, is located one to three inches inside the vagina directly over the urethra, at the neck of the bladder. Often, during G-spot stimulation, women will sense the urge to pee and if this spot is stimulated too aggressively, you may be left feeling like you're peeing fire or razorblades afterwards. Now, I don't know about you, but the feeling of fiery razor blades sliding down the urethral shaft after intercourse does not bring warm fuzzies to mind (or body). Additionally, the inside vaginal wall, where the G-spot is located, has significantly fewer nerve endings, compared to other vulvar tissues, which makes it more difficult to have an orgasm with direct G-spot stimulation and/or through penile thrusting. Due to this fact and the likely potential of irritating the urethra, most women wave the white flag long before they are able to reach their climax. But don't get too disappointed, there are other "spots" that produce the same glorious response as the intended G-spot.

Let's start with one of the easiest "spots" to identify and to stimulate, termed the U-spot. No courtship required here! Direct and persistent, but gentle, stimulation over the U-spot is like a soothing bath after a long stressful day. Rhythmic circles, stroking or vibration to this spot further heightens the sensations and facilitates true euphoria. The U-spot is found just above, next to, or slightly diagonally up (depending on the individual anatomy) from the urethral opening. This spot is actually where the Skene's glands are located and has contractile tissue which aids in the production of an orgasm (See Figure 3).

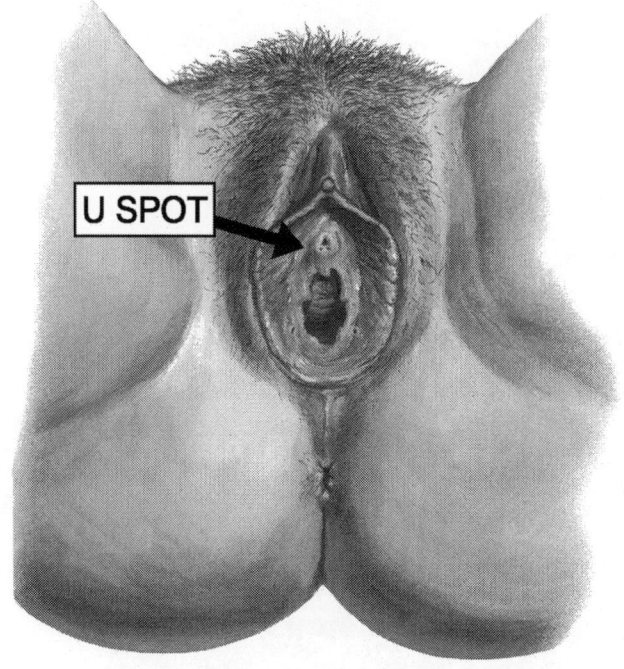

Figure 3

In fact, the U-spot orgasm can produce such deep uterine contractions, it will have your entire body leaping, gyrating and quivering right off the bed. This is a spot every man should know about because it serves as a great starting point for female arousal.

The next spot is termed the A-spot, or the Anterior Fornix Erogenous spot. This is a little more tricky to find, but is known for producing instant vaginal lubrication and pleasant, but intense, deep orgasms. Unfortunately, men practically have to be an anatomist to locate this little pleasure place. The A-spot is hidden just anterior to the cervix (see Figure 4) between the uterus and the bladder. The other location for this A-spot is actually posterior to the cervix between the uterus and the rectum (see Figure 4).

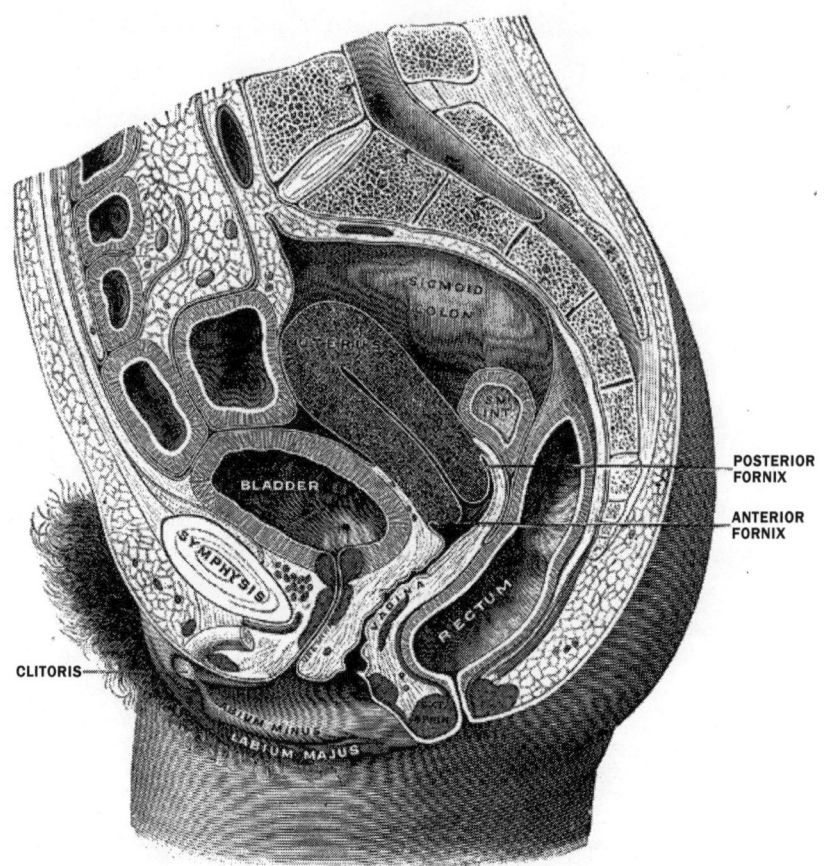

Figure 4

Due to the close proximity of the bladder (if going anteriorly) and the rectum (if going posteriorly) during stimulation, this A-spot is not very high on the popularity list. If this spot is not stimulated accurately, you may feel an uncomfortable pressure against your bladder or rectum. This may become a problem if you are trying to get lost in the moment of arousal and orgasmic bliss. If so, don't worry, for many goers it's often not too successful with the first few attempts. However, you may find that a little coaching and patience could prove this spot to be an exciting trinket of happiness.

The last, but certainly not least, "spot" of orgasmic satisfaction is the clitoris. As discussed earlier, the clitoris is located at the apex of the vulva with thousands of nerve endings ready to respond to the slightest of touch. Like the other three spots previously mentioned, there are a few pros and cons of clitoral stimulation that one should know. The clitoris is easy to identify and easy to access. For most women, it's the "go-to" spot that will produce an orgasm with nearly every attempt. It has a remarkable ability to produce intense, fast-achieving superficial orgasms (clitoral stimulated clitoral orgasms) and deep, lasting pelvic floor orgasms (clitoral stimulated vaginal orgasms). The thousands of nerve endings located here help generate heightened and lingering sensations, as well as the ability to create multiple orgasmic experiences. However, these nerve endings may also produce and be responsible for pain during intercourse, particularly if approached too quickly or too aggressively. Additionally, if the clitoris is stimulated for an extended period of time without achieving the goal of orgasm, it may become temporarily desensitized and feel numb. When this happens, it is not likely the clitoris will produce an orgasm. Don't worry, this is typically a short-lived response and will wear off with rest and time.

It's important to know where these "hot" spots are on your body and how aroused, if at all, you are when they are stimulated. One reason many women can achieve multiple orgasms is because there are typically multiple places that can bring her to climax. The possibilities are many. The potential is high. The first step is to explore these areas and discover what works for you. Remember, not every women responds the same way. Some need a little and some need a lot. With your husband, finding out what takes you to ultimate gratification should be rewarding and exciting.

CHAPTER FOUR

Handle With Care...And Your Vagina Will Thank You For It!

Caring for your vagina seems like an easy enough task for the average girl. I mean, you've been doing it your whole life. There's nothing to it, right? Well, there are some common mistakes that we, as women, do to our vaginas every day. Unknowingly, we put ourselves at higher risk for infection, vaginal irritation and/or vulvar pain. However, with a few adjustments, you can see significant changes in the way your body, particularly the vagina, feels and looks.

Let's start with vaginal hygiene. Many women have anxiety or fears about mild odors and/or discharge that come from their vaginas. Often, it's a natural, harmless aspect of cyclical hormonal changes or foods we eat that creates this mild odor that can be perceived as unpleasant. I'm not talking about white, clumpy or yellow/green discharge that has a significantly foul odor. That would definitely earn you a trip to the gynecologist. The odor I'm referring to is what most women would refer to as a "musty smell". As a result of this natural odor, many women scrub the daylights out of their vaginas in hopes to rid their bodies of the scent. In actuality, soap should never be used between the labia or inside the vagina. Not soap, not douching, not cleaning cloths or feminine wipes, nada. We are self-cleaning ovens, Ladies. All we need is water. When you are in the shower, separate the labia and allow water to rinse you and you're clean.

When we use soap in between the labia and/or inside the vagina, we can induce several negative things to our vaginas. First, and most commonly, we can create vaginal dryness. Vaginal dryness can lead to tissue fragility and, thus, increased risk for painful intercourse. Second, we can change the pH in the vaginal canal and create a breeding ground for bacteria to grow. Bad bacteria, if introduced repeatedly, may be difficult to get rid of and can become a chronic problem. Finally, using soap in this delicately balanced area can wash the normal, healthy bacteria out of our vaginas which, again, set us up for potential infections. And let's face it, Ladies, men never prep for sex. They've touched their penis 10,000 times a day to adjust it, pee, make sure it's still there, adjust, and so on. They've handled money, shook the neighbor's hand, made a sandwich, opened doors, picked their noses, etc. all the while touching their penis throughout the day to make sure it hasn't left their bodies unexpectedly. When it's time to have sex, they don't take time to wash their penises. Most of the time, they are just excited that the time has arrived! All the while, WE, with our hang-ups about odors, are cleansing our vaginas with Vanilla Bean and Lavender soap to prepare for sex, washing our own healthy bacteria out, just to introduce his inside. Stop the madness, Ladies. Simply use water and you're clean. (Side note: This does not include your anus. You can use soap there.)

Some of you may be asking, "What about after having sex?" "How do I get the lube off?" "What can I do to decrease my risks of infections?" The answer lies in a simple, but effective, formula. After having intercourse, take a wet wash cloth and wipe the vulva/vagina front to back. Fold the cloth a time or two more and repeat. In fact, any time you are cleaning the vulva/vagina, for instance after you pee, you should always wipe front to back. This will help prevent bacteria from going up into the urethra. The second half of this formula is simply put, "Pee Before and Pee After." Empty your bladder before you have sex, so that the penis doesn't push against a full bladder, and pee a little after you have sex....even if just a little tinkle comes out. The acidity from the urine will help kill any bacteria that the penis, or hands, has introduced during your rendezvous.

Another way to decrease your risk of infection is choosing the right lubrication. First, before we go any further, I believe every woman should use lubrication whenever she's planning to have intercourse. Even if you think you're the fountain of youth "down there," use it! We, women, have the amazing ability to produce good lubrication during anticipation and arousal, however, we also have the ability to dry up rather, and surprisingly, quickly. We can be completely engaged and into the moment while having sex with our husbands and then, out of the blue, our minds to go into multitasking mode. "Did we pick up the laundry from the dry cleaners?" "Did I start the dishwasher?" "Did the kids do their homework?" "Why is he grunting like that?" That's all it takes, and all the natural moisture (we were so proud of) dries up like the Sahara Desert. When you're dry, you are almost guaranteed to have painful intercourse. One episode of pain with intercourse sets you up for MANY episodes of pain. Why? Because your vagina has a good memory and will close up shop if she's had a bad experience.

Clearly, lubrication is a necessity and plays an important role for future sexual encounters you'll have with your husband. Did you also know that certain types of lubrication can actually be harmful to vaginal tissues and cause discomfort during intercourse? Many of the water-based and silicone lubrications out on the market, which are readily available at major grocery chains, have glycerin in them. Glycerin is a sugar. A sugar in a nice, warm, wet environment has a high potential to grow yeast. Perhaps that is where your recurrent yeast infections are coming from. My recommendations? Olive oil or coconut oil. I know, I know, it's not so romantic to have the economy size olive oil container awaiting on the night stand, but it's a fabulous lubricant!...and, per ounce, is cheaper! I also like coconut oil for its antifungal, antibacterial and antimicrobial properties. And, if you are a germ-a-phobe like me, you can rest at ease when you coat the penis with this gem of a lubricant. Both lubricants are completely safe to use and typically don't need any reapplying during a single love-making session.

Be sure to coat the penis well with lubricant. Most women think, "Well, I'm the one with the dryness. I should put this on me." However, it will do more good for you to apply the lubricant to his penis. Be generous with the lubricant and coat the entire shaft of the penis. Believe me, he won't mind at all. This is foreplay for him. A little heed of warning, though, if you use olive oil and get a little crazy when applying it to the penis, it WILL stain your sheets, it's OIL. Here's a little tip: you can protect your bedding by putting a dark colored towel underneath you. Again, there is no need for you to try to scrub the olive or coconut oil out of your vagina. Simply use the washcloth with the front to back cleansing method, then pee afterwards and you'll be good to go!

Another important aspect of vaginal hygiene and risk management for vaginal infections involves your pubic hair. For the past several years, the latest craze in vaginal hygiene is to remove all of the pubic hair, either by a Brazilian wax or shaving with a razor blade. Somehow, this hairless phenomenon is becoming the social "norm" and considered sexy. As if coating the outside of your labia with hot, dripping wax and ripping the hair from its roots (in sections!!!) doesn't sound horrible enough, let me give you some good reasons why pubic hair is a must.

Pubic hair keeps unwanted germs away. The hair is thought to act as a passive protective barrier against bacteria that you might pick up from a toilet seat or your hands. This has not been clinically researched, merely hypothesized; however, it seems reasonable. Other reasons that may have you putting down the razor blade include potential skin irritation, cuts and nicks, damage to hair follicles, ingrown hairs and vulvar itching and/or burning. When you remove the hair, you are leaving the tissue exposed for infection and/or injury. With that said, let me encourage you to leave some hair over the labia, at minimal, and trim around the bikini lines if you wish.

So to recap, when it comes to sex, no prepping is necessary (unless you've just finished working out). Resist the urge to use soaps, lotions, feminine wipes and/or douches. Leave a little hair over the labial major to decrease your risk of potential infection and be sure to use the correct lubrication during intercourse (olive oil, coconut oil or glycerin free water based lubricants). Using the wrong kind of lube can increase your risk for infections. Whenever you are cleaning up "down there," be consistent at wiping in a front to back motion. Finally, always remember to pee before and pee after.

CHAPTER 5

The Big "O": Why Can't I Have One?

As promised, the time has come to unveil the secrets behind The Big "O", the orgasm. The orgasm is unique and intensely satisfying. It is medically defined as a sudden discharge of accumulated sexual tension during the sexual response cycle, resulting in rhythmic muscular contractions of the pelvic floor muscles and is characterized by intense sensations of pleasure. Essentially, peaked sexual stimulation and arousal will eventually lead to spontaneous muscle contractions and ecstasy. Its ability to facilitate involuntary body movement and fascial expressions makes it nearly impossible to deny when experienced. Yet many women do not experience an orgasm regularly or at all.

The latest research surveys reveal that 25% of women always have an orgasm during sexual encounters (for men it's 90%). In other words, the majorities of women are NOT experiencing, or have never experienced, intense orgasmic pleasure during intimacy. Very few women, less than 10%, have a medical condition that inhibits their ability to have an orgasm at all, but that's a small percentage in the large scheme of things. So what's the story for the rest of the sexually, unsatisfied women? It's a problem that has gained a lot of media attention off and on throughout the years, but more recently has raised a lot of concerns.

In an article entitled *Female Orgasm May Be Tied to 'Rule of Thumb',* which was later publicized by abcnews.com, sexuality researchers explained if men and women knew their biology (i.e. their sexual anatomy), their sex lives might improve. One researcher continues by saying,

> "What is startling and surprising to me is that both men and women buy into the same sort of cultural model," he said. "If he is a good lover, he can bring me to orgasm with his penis alone. And a man buys into that and doesn't offer any kind of stimulation. And because he's not any good, she won't say anything because it's emasculating." "We need to know how to talk about sex and communicate about what feels good and not be so scared."

Hence, the reason for this book! Researcher, Elisabeth Lloyd, a professor of history, philosophical science and biology at the Indiana University and is best known for her extensive study on sex and the female orgasm, agrees and adds that too much emphasis is placed on models of female sexuality that are created by Hollywood and the pornography industry. Believe it or not, besides the fact that pornography is completely scripted and a pathetic representation of a healthy sexual relationship, it is created BY men FOR men. As a result, skewed thinking on behalf of men AND women regarding how sex should be significantly interferes with a woman's ability to have an orgasm. So, what is one to do? Well, knowledge is power! And power, in this case, is PLEASURE!

Here's what we know. Most women do not orgasm with penile penetration alone. <*Sigh of relief*> Most women do not orgasm with each sexual encounter (a statistic that is sure to improve by the end of this book). Most men are unaware of what needs to take place for a woman's mind and body to have an orgasm (another statistic that we hope to change). By now, you may be asking yourself so what DOES have to take place to have an orgasm? There are actually a group of processes that must transpire in order for an orgasm to occur. These processes, consisting of arousal, stimulation, climax and relaxation, can be defined as the "sexual response cycle". All four stages of this response cycle are necessary and important in the climatic experience.

The sexual response cycle consists of an excitement phase, plateau phase, orgasmic phase and resolution phase. Each phase plays an essential role in sexual intimacy and requires its own careful attention. In some cases, practicing skills in one phase may help you achieve and reach other phases more regularly and quickly. Such is the case with the excitement phase.

Excitement Phase: This excitement phase has the ability to make or break your experience. This phase has limitless possibilities for you and your lover. It has the potential to be the most creative and fun of all the phases combined. During the excitement phase, erogenous zones are teased and flirted with and your five senses are perking up. This phase is what we typically call "foreplay" and, for women, it includes physical AND mental arousal. Because this phase includes mental preparation and anticipation about your sexy, love encounter, it has the potential to start hours (and sometimes days) before you enter your boudoir. Receiving and sending exotic love letters, emails, phone calls or texts to your husband or buying sexy clothing or underwear help to moisten the taste buds for what's to come.

During the excitement phase, create your own sexy environment. As discussed earlier, this may include music, flowers, candles, lingerie, etc. Force yourself to let go of the day's heightened events or stresses. If you need a bubble bath to do this, then so be it. Start meditating on all the things you enjoy about your spouse and sex (remember the "confirmation bias" principle), even if it's been awhile since you've had a positive experience with intercourse. Play your own little fantasy about you and your hubby in your mind; how he might kiss you or gently stroke your bare skin with his fingertips. Gently squeeze the pelvic floor muscles in short, pulses to facilitate blood flow to the labia (I call this "priming the pump").

When it's time to come together, take your time and don't give into anxiety about rushing to the next step. Allow yourself to be the "Giver" and the "Receiver" during mutual stimulation and arousal. Gently guide your spouse and educate him on what feels good. Men really would prefer to know. However, be sure not to ruin the moment with a long lecture or sharp interjection about how he's missing your "spot". Simply give him a sign or verbal gesture of pleasure when he's there. Guide his hand or use his penis to help him explore your body. Trust me; he'll catch on really fast.

During this excitement phase, the vaginal tissues become alert, the clitoris more erect and the muscles start building in tension. The nipples will start to protrude and the face, neck and chest will flush. With continued stimulation of arousal zones (i.e. vulvar tissues, nipples, neck, inner thighs, abdomen), the heart rate increases, the breath quickens and a warming sensation begins to rise up from within. You may also notice increased vaginal lubrication, a little or a lot depending on your current hormonal levels. This phase typically last several minutes to hours, depending on how much time you are investing in the preparations.

Most of the time, if you don't get this part, you won't progress to an orgasm or you may view your sexual encounter as very dissatisfying and unfulfilling. The fact is, most women never get to this phase or perhaps they reach this phase for a few minutes before their mate is rushing to the next phase or completing his orgasm. And, oh, by the way, sex does not have to end after his climax, particularly if he jumps the boat too quickly. Now, if you intensify this excitement phase, you'll move quickly to the next phase, Plateau Phase.

Plateau Phase: I like to describe this phase as one who puts their car in neutral and presses on the accelerator. All the sensations from the excitement phase are revving up, ready with potential to take off (more like explode) at any moment. All the physical signs seen during the excitement phase are now more pronounced and deepened. The vagina continues to swell from increased blood flow and the clitoris becomes very hypersensitive, even to the point of pain for some women, so be careful. If the clitoris becomes painful for you, try stimulating a different spot, such as the U-spot, nipples or another erotic place on your body so there is no interruption of built up sexual excitement.

During the plateau phase, muscle tension will continue to grow and intensify, and not just in the pelvic floor. You may notice muscle tension in your feet, hands, arms and face….which would explain all the funny faces you (or your partner) make. At any point during the excitement phase or the plateau phase, this sexual tension and arousal can come to a screeching halt. And it doesn't take much. We women are really bad about this. If we are not careful, we can allow our minds to wander, become annoyed by a sound or interrupted by the children. Children, by the way, win the award for being the number one killers of libido. They seem to have a sixth sense when it comes to parental intimacy. They may have a perfect five year history of sleeping through the night, but the night you choose to make it extra spicy and sexy; they will knock on the door asking for a glass of water. With the exception of the children, you can help avoid this unwanted interruption.

If you allow it, your mind with wander to various events or unresolved situations of your day which will, in turn, successfully pull you out of the plateau phase. And you NEED the plateau phase to get you to orgasmic phase. So, help yourself out with what I call "mental narration". As you are engaging in sexiness with your lover, write a love novel in your mind about WHAT he's doing to you AS he is doing it. Be as graphic as you wish as you narrate how he is kissing you and where he's touching your body. Make note of your response, the warmth rising up within you, moistened vagina and how it makes you feel so good. Don't be modest or embarrassed with your descriptions, after all, it is a love novel about you and your spouse! Practicing mental narration will help keep your mind focused on your spouse as well as contribute to your sexual tension that's preparing you for orgasm.

Orgasmic Phase: The ultimate goal of sexual pleasure is the orgasm. This is the shortest of all the phases, but most gratifying. Once you've hit this phase, there is no turning back. In other words, you can't be in this phase and decide to delay your climax or turn back. When you're there, you're there and it *will* happen. Ironically, this phase is not just a continuation of the first two phases. One additional component must be added during your sexual climb in order to achieve The Big "O" and it's found in the brain. I know, it's the brain thing again!

In the early 2000s, researchers from the University of Groningen in the Netherlands did a sexy little study where they look at people's brains *while* they were being sexually stimulated by their partners. *Yeah...I know! Talk about being a fly on the wall!* What they found was what we knew all along. Women have to feel safe and secure in order to reach climax. In other words, the part of the brain that harbors worry, anxiety and fear must be shut off in order to have an orgasm. This sounds like a no-brainer (no pun intended), but women are not good at this at all! For most women, this may come in the form of anxiety about being too fat or how you look with the lights on or fear about being hurt (as seen with chronic vaginal dryness or pelvic pain, for example). As mentioned previously, there is help for this by way of a physician, women's health physical therapist and/or sex therapist/psychologist. So don't settle for the idea that you can't have an orgasm or it's too much work. *(Side note: Please keep in mind, antidepressants/anxiety, blood pressure and allergy medications can inhibit your ability to achieve an orgasm. Discuss options with your physician before stopping or adjusting these medications.)* Figure out what you need to let your guard down, turning off all fear and anxiety, and let your orgasm take control.

When your brain and body are in alignment for climatic bliss, the sexual tension that has been building up during the first two phases will be powerfully liberated. During this time, your heart rate and breathing are at their highest rates and, for most, muscles will begin to contract more rapidly in the vagina, uterus, abdomen and feet. Red blotchy patches, which are harmless areas of increased blood flow, will appear over your body, most visibly seen on the face, ears, neck, breast and back. This reaction occurs in all phases of the sexual response cycle, but is most apparent during the orgasmic phase. It is known as the "sex flush". *This is why it's quite obvious that you weren't just "taking a nap" on a Sunday afternoon.*

The orgasmic phase typically lasts 10-20 seconds for women and is much shorter in duration for men. The orgasm is unique in that it facilitates involuntary muscle contractions throughout the body while releasing bonding and relaxation hormones in the brain. Masters and Johnson, who dedicated their entire careers to the study human sexuality, found that men took an average of 4 minutes to reach orgasm with their partners whereas women took 10-20 minutes with their partners. However, when women masturbated in private, it took them 4 minutes or less. Why, you ask? Because women were able to turn off their defense mechanisms easily when they were in private. I illustrate this finding to emphasize the importance of releasing fear and anxiety when engaging in sexual intimacy with your spouse. It's crucial for a healthy, fulfilling sex life and, in my opinion, a prime reason for a sexless marriage.

Resolution Phase: The resolution phase is known as the recovery phase. It is here, that the body will return to its' status quo. The heart rate and breathing slow down and all the erect tissues retreat to their normal resting place. Vaginal swelling and muscular tension will ease and become relaxed. Your reddened tissues will return to normal color. Due to the release of oxytocin, vasopressin and dopamine in the brain, partners will feel a sense of gratification, bonding and relaxation after orgasm.

During the resolution phase, men and women may, or may not, go into a refractory period, or a waiting period. The refractory period is marked by the inability or intolerance for continued sexual stimulation due to genital hypersensitivity/pain and/or fatigue. Men frequently enter the refractory period for an unspecified length of time. This time varies from human to human and increases with age. Women, however, typically have a much shorter refractory period, or none at all, and will fall back into plateau phase. Therefore, further stimulation will produce additional orgasms. Women are much more likely to have multiple orgasms than our counterparts. *Yeah for us!* However, with practice, men can learn to have multiple orgasms with significantly shorter refractory periods.

So, as you can see, the phases of the sexual response cycle are necessary when it comes to having The Big "O" experience. Perhaps the reason you haven't had an orgasm, or not in the past 10 years, is because each individual phase has not been explored or respected. It's important to know what each phase consists of so that you can make adjustments in your own sexual life. Remember, each woman is different and will experience sexual intimacy uniquely. So, don't force yourself into a box rather use this knowledge as a guideline to maximize your potential!

CHAPTER SIX

What's Going On Down There? When Things Are Just NOT Feeling Right

The mood is right. The lights are low. The environment is saturated with sexual possibilities. You are fully expecting to make this night a better-than-our-usual sex night. You've pulled out, more like dusted off, the lingerie you wore when you were first married and misted yourself lightly with your favorite perfume. You even "committed" yourself earlier in the day by flirting with your husband about how you planned to make him smile later on that evening. You're ready, he's ready. The time is right and the process begins to unfold.

However, soon after things get started, something doesn't feel right. Something is pinching or pulling at you in all the wrong places. You blame the fasteners on your sex-goddess lingerie and try to push past the discomfort. But this time, it's not that easy. The discomfort is steadily increasing until all you can do is close your eyes tightly and hope that he has a sudden onset of premature ejaculation. You wince in pain and pull out your white flag in surrender. And just like that, your sexy night is over before it even began. You're disappointment resounds like a symphony in a concert hall and all you're left with are questions and, of course, a very sore vagina.

Believe it or not, this is a common scenario that shakes the very foundation of many women. It affects more than 30% of women in the United States. This figure does not account for women who have *not* sought out medical help/treatment for their very intimate and, in many cases, embarrassing pain. It's incidences like this that have the potential to unravel the very fabric of a solid marriage. Believe it or not, many women experience, or have experienced, pain and/or discomfort during sexual intimacy beginning unexpectedly as described above. The onset of vaginal pain during intercourse does not have to be linked to any history of sexual abuse or fear about having sex. Although, these kinds of things will affect your ability to engage in and enjoy sexual intimacy. However, that is not the case for the majority. There is quite a large population of women experiencing pain during intercourse who have no prior history of abuse or injury. Statistics shows that approximately 1 in 3 women have or have experienced pelvic pain during intercourse in their lifetime. Additionally, research shows that women will seek an average of 7 doctors, including specialists, to receive one diagnosis of pelvic pain. In fact, pelvic pain, and/or pain during intercourse, is the number two complaint at a gynecologist's office. However, due to the complexity of pelvic and vaginal pain, it is extremely difficult to diagnose and even more tricky to treat. For decades, physicians have tried traditional medical treatments for pelvic pain included numbing ointments/creams, oral medications and vaginal surgery or hysterectomy. Unfortunately, more times than not, if a medical professional cannot find the source of your vaginal pain and is unsuccessful at curing you, they often turf you off for a psychological evaluation and/or suggest that your pain is "all in your mind". In fact, for decades women have been told to "have a glass of wine and lube up" or "have sex in the bathtub" in order to have comfortable sex. Really?!?! Have sex in the bathtub?!?! First of all, why must a woman intoxicate herself in order to have pain-free sex. And, secondly, whose bathtub is big enough to have sex in anyways! Let's not forget to mention the fact that you increase your risk for infections and you lose all natural lubrication when having sex in water. Although, these treatments and recommendations are typically made with good intentions, they frequently do not produce favorable results, if any.

Does one episode of painful intercourse mean that you now HAVE pelvic pain? No, but it has the potential to create a full-size, on-going problem! Remember, your vagina has a really good memory and if she is hurt during one sexual encounter, she is more likely to experience pain and/or discomfort for many encounters to come. It is as if, when meeting someone for the first time, you extend your hand in a friendly greeting only to receive a sucker punch to the gut instead. The next time you see that individual, you will most likely brace and guard yourself from a second punch. But, imagine, if this happened every time you saw that person. You will most likely not be relaxed and inviting when they walk in the room. And so it goes with your vagina. The more you open yourself for sexual intimacy that ends in pain, the more likely it will be painful the next go around. Unless, of course, something breaks the pain cycle.

So what makes the vagina hurt? We've discussed a few contributory factors already such as hormonal imbalance, chronic vaginal dryness, inadequate or inappropriate lubrication and/or poor libido. However, even if all of these factors are working as they should, you could still have pain or discomfort during intercourse. "Why?" you ask. Because there are other things to consider "down-there" that can make or break a sexual encounter. These "things" are some of the primary reasons pelvic pain is so difficult to diagnose and the reason why women who *are* diagnosed differ in symptoms and intensities of pain. Some women may feel itchy and/or burning, while others feel sharp and/or stabbing. Still others may experience lower abdominal cramping, urinary retention or urgency whereas others have low back pain and constipation. All these symptoms can intermingle and fluctuate in severity from day to day. Take note, the longer the symptoms last, the more difficult it is to identify its origin and effectively treat.

The truth is, the multifaceted dynamics of pelvic pain, in itself, puzzles most healthcare professionals today. Most patients are often left feeling discouraged or hopeless after visiting their doctors. With few reliable and credible pelvic pain resources available, patients often turn to the internet for education and/or treatment suggestions. Now we all know there is a lot of sketchy, unreliable information that pops up on the internet when performing a search, particularly if you are not familiar with the field or specialty. An inexperienced web searcher may become horrified when stumbling upon a blog of someone's accidental surgical/medical botches that left her disfigured or in worse pain. Therefore, to save you the agony of misrepresentation of information, I will discuss typical scenarios that contribute to pelvic pain and, *of course*, painful intercourse.

Pelvic pain typically involves the pelvic floor musculature, surrounding nerves and pelvic organs, commonly the bladder and/or rectum. Each involved area should be appropriately evaluated when determining the origin of the pain because sometimes dysfunction in one area can be linked to pain in a different area. Such is the case with bladder pain, for example. Greater than 90% of patients with Interstitial Cystitis, or Painful Bladder Syndrome, also have pelvic floor muscles spasms or dysfunction. However, it is not known which of these things came first. Is the bladder pain causing the pelvic floor muscle spasms/dysfunction or are the spasms/dysfunction causing the bladder pain? Nonetheless, we **do** know that it is rare to see one without the other and attempting to treat one without consideration of the other is not wise. Another example of this phenomenon is demonstrated with bowel dysfunctions. At times, when the deeper pelvic floor muscles go into spasms or are chronically in a shortened position, one may experience severe rectal pain, anal stenosis (narrowing of the anal canal), rectal pressure and/or constipation.

Let's dissect further the reasons one might have painful intercourse. The one common denominator of the above examples is the involvement of the musculoskeletal system, primarily *(but not limited to)* the pelvic floor muscles. Remember from previous chapters, you learned that the pelvic floor muscles are responsible for relaxing enough to allow penile entry as well as producing rhythmic muscular contractions that progressively intensify to generate an orgasm. If these muscles are too spastic (i.e. too tight) or have trigger points within the muscle belly (i.e. muscular knots, if you will), then these muscles may not have the ability to relax enough for the penis to enter. Also, if the penis happens to find its way through the restricted vaginal opening *(which it has the most remarkable ability to do)*, then it may produce a raw, ripping or knife-life sensation. Additionally, occasionally these "knots" in the muscles make it very difficult, or even inhibit, for the muscles to contract and relax quickly during stimulation. As a result, sometimes, even without vaginal penetration, just having an orgasm can be painful during and/or afterwards. This may present itself in the form of a deep pelvic ache, rectal pain, and/or clitoral or vulvar stinging, itching or burning. The pelvic floor muscles are not typically the only culprit that can wreak this kind of havoc on the body. Accessory muscles can also become problematic, as well.

Common accessory muscles that also contribute to painful intercourse consist of the abdominals, hip adductors (i.e. inner thigh muscles), lower back, gluteals (i.e. buttocks) and external rotators (i.e. deep hip muscles that allow the knee and foot to rotate inward or outward). With individuals who suffer with pelvic pain, these muscles frequently have muscular trigger points and/or tension. These trigger points and muscular tension often builds up from chronic, static positions or repetitive movements that our bodies endure everyday as seen with, *oh, let's say,* prolonged sitting at a desk job, poor body mechanics during housecleaning, carrying the kids on one hip or standing on tile floor without proper supportive shoes for hours at a time…like those cute, red pumps that make your calves look iron man (*I can't think of ANY woman that does that! Wink, wink*). I could go on to tell you how these muscular trigger points can lay along the same fascial planes of the pelvic floor muscles which will result in abnormal tensile forces going through the pelvis when activated, or how the referral pain pattern for most of these accessory muscles travel to the vagina or rectum, but I will save you the technical agony. Here's what you need to know. When you're lying on your back, with your legs open, ready for sexiness to happen, these trigger points can become activated and/or muscles can become over-stretched causing referral pain to the vagina during intercourse.

Muscles are not the only thing that can cause pelvic pain during intercourse. The nerves going through those muscles can be troublesome, too. These nerve endings can become quenched from muscular tension, entangled in connective tissue or even entrapped from surgical mesh placed during organ prolapse surgery (*which is a big topic in the news today due to the significant volume of women reporting post-operative complications from the synthetic mesh*). Individuals with this type of problem will typically feel severe pain during sitting, numbness and/or tingling in the groin or down the leg. This can lead to debilitating pain in the vagina or rectum, create urinary incontinence and/or, *you guessed it*, pain during intercourse. The vaginal pain from intercourse will typically be noticed upon initial penetration, but can also be facilitated with deep thrusting. The pain is described as sharp, stabbing, shooting, cutting and/or electrifying with referral sites of pain to the inner thigh, vagina, rectum, buttocks, clitoris and/or the bladder. These individuals feel much better sitting on a toilet seat rather than a chair because it decompresses the nerve. Nerve pain typically loves ice. Therefore, ice applied to the perineum, the space between the vaginal opening and anus, may temporarily ease pudendal nerve discomfort. If you are headed for the freezer right now, please be sure to place a soft cloth or towel between you and the ice pack and apply for no more than 20 minutes at a time.

Visceral, or organ, problems can also create pain during intercourse. The most common of diagnoses that fall in this category are endometriosis and interstitial cystitis, a.k.a. I.C. or Painful Bladder Syndrome. Most women are familiar with the term endometriosis because more likely than not, she knows someone who has had it or has experienced it herself. It is defined as the growth of endometrial cells (cells that normally line the uterus wall) outside of the uterus. These cells can be found on the cervix, ovaries, fallopian tubes, the bladder, rectum, pelvic cavity and/or attached to the bowels. The strange thing about endometriosis is that severity of the condition does not correlate to the severity of pain. In other words, some women can be filled with endometriosis and not have any pain while others suffer excruciating pain and have small amounts of endometriosis. Endo pain is typically cyclic, but pain with intercourse caused from endometriosis adhesions are not. Women with endometriosis will experience pain during intercourse more often than pain-free intercourse. Often endo pain can be relieved by reducing trigger points found in the pelvic floor musculature and abdomen, as well as visceral mobilization techniques to free up restrictions.

While endometriosis is a well-known and understood disease, interstitial cystitis is certainly not. Interstitial cystitis is a poorly understood pathology involving the bladder and/or the urethra characterized by one or more of the following symptoms: bladder and/or urethral pain during urination, urgency and frequency, bladder spasms, lower abdominal cramping, urinary retention, voiding hesitancy, pain with bladder filling and/or urinary incontinence (*just to name a few*). An individual can present with one or more of these above symptoms which can be constant or intermittent in severity. Individuals with Painful Bladder Syndrome will often describe their pain in terms of "flares" and are able to pinpoint certain "triggers" which provoke their symptoms.

There are several leading hypothesis about what causes interstitial cystitis in individuals. These theories include the presence of low level bacteria that is resistant to antibiotics and/or goes undetected by urinalysis, the abnormal trigger of Mast cells (inflammatory cells) that get released into the bladder, damage to the bladder's protective inner layer which allows irritating urine contents to penetrate the lining, and, lastly, pelvic floor muscular tension (spasms and/or trigger points and/or myofascial restrictions) that can cause nerve irritability, referral pain and the release of inflammation in the bladder. Again, there is currently not a concrete answer to which of these factors cause I.C., but we know for sure that the majority of women also have pelvic floor tension and myofascial restrictions.

It is also very common to have bowel dysfunction, such as Irritable Bowel Syndrome (or IBS) or Inflammatory Bowel Disease (IBD) along with interstitial cystitis. This is due to the shared nerve fibers and/or connections between the organs. However, other contributing factors include increased psychological stress from having a chronic pain condition, and the presence of high inflammatory markers typically found in affected individuals. Women with IBS and/or IBD may not be able to tolerate deep penetration from their partners or simply the weight of their partner's body against their abdomen. Orgasms may also create or lead to cramping in their lower abdomen which could, in turn, provoke an onset of bowel symptoms.

Certain autoimmune pathologies can also lead to dysfunctions/disorders of the musculoskeletal, visceral or neuropathic systems causing pain during intercourse, poor bladder and/or bowel control or inadequate pelvic organ support. Some of these conditions include, but are not limited to, Fibromyalgia, Multiple Sclerosis, Systemic Lupus Erythematosus, Parkinson's disease, Ehlers-Danlos Syndrome, Hashimoto's Disease and other thyroid disorders, Rheumatoid Arthritis, Addison's Disease, etc. Adequate and skilled management of these pathologies is the key to improving the quality of intimacy with your significant other.

Whether the origin of pain is musculoskeletal, neurological or visceral in nature, many of these problems can be treated conservatively and quite successfully. You do not have to live with or even "tolerate" painful intercourse. There are actual healthcare providers that specialize in pelvic pain and pelvic floor disorders. They are very familiar with and treat these problems every day. We are one of them! At Women First Rehabilitation, some of the primary diagnoses we evaluate and treat are pelvic pain and pain during intercourse. We work closely with the patient's existing medical provider(s) to ensure that each patient is able to maximize their potential of healing. It is our belief that skilled pelvic floor rehabilitation, along with adequate medical management, offers the most success for alleviating painful intercourse and restoring intimacy. However, not all healthcare professionals are created equal, so do your homework and do not settle for just any old provider. Find one who is willing to stick it out with you.

CHAPTER SEVEN

What Are My Options? Treatment and Management for Painful Intercourse

Part 1: Treatment Choices

So now that you know that painful intercourse can be treated successfully, take a moment to sigh with relief. Painful intercourse may be tricky and very complex, but it is NOT impossible to treat. The most difficult part of the entire healing process is finding someone (or a team of "someones") skilled enough, persistent enough and willing to do the job. As mentioned before, women will go to an average of 7-10 doctors before receiving one diagnosis regarding their pelvic or vaginal pain. And even when they do get a diagnosis, the health care provider, independently, has a limited bag of "tools" to offer patients as help. After all the creams, jellys, salves, oral medication, injections, and, yes, surgeries have failed, patients are often left feeling like freaks of nature who cannot be helped…a very sad scenario that happens to thousands of patients every day.

Is the physician bad? Are his or her techniques incorrect? Are they just trying to throw something at you to get you to go away?

The answer is a resounding No, No and No *(in most cases)*. Most physicians are using the very best of their ability and knowledge to heal you and to DO NO HARM (from their Hippocratic Oath). The problem isn't the physician; it is the lack of teamwork and fluidity within the medical community; as well as, the innocent ignorance and, perhaps, inexperience with pelvic pain. There are so few health care professionals that treat these kinds of problems; it's often difficult to locate other disciplines that effectively treat pelvic pain and related disorders. If I may sound like a broken record for a second, *pelvic pain is most successfully treated when a team of providers are connected by communicating with each other, trusting in the other's ability to contribute to the healing process and willing to work with each other without feeling threatened or offended by another specialty.* Sounds simple enough? Well it's not. Let me illustrate this point with an example patient. This is a common story that is retold by countless women that I treat in my practice every day.

Marcia is a 23 yr old female who has been in an unconsummated marriage for the past 10 months. She went to her gynecologist who, after prescribing numbing jelly and vaginal hormones (which failed), decided that her pain is coming from the inability to relax "down there" due to fear and/or avoidance. *Here it comes*, "Have a glass of wine and use lots of lube," he says, "You just need to relax a little. It's all in your mind." When this doesn't work, she doesn't even bother going back because she feels demeaned, dismissed and degraded. She decides to try another physician. This time, she chooses a female gynecologist because "females know best." The new physician tries a number of birth control pills, bioidentical hormone replacements and several steroid injections directly into the fragile vulvar tissues, but Marcia gets no relief of her symptoms. Feeling desperate to help Marcia, she suggests an exploratory laparoscopic procedure revealing minimal to moderate evidence of endometriosis which is properly removed. This, however, does not cure Marcia's problem with painful intercourse. Her new physician looks up the name of a sex therapist, sadly informs Marcia that she has done all she can do and turfs her off for a psych consult. Marcia, feeling hopeless and frustrated from all the failed treatment, decides to go to the sex therapist for help. After all, her new marriage *is* suffering from the lack of intimacy and quite frankly, she doesn't even desire her husband as she once did. Several months of sex therapy, with prescribed abstinence, does the trick to boost Marcia's spirits and encourages her to give sex another try. So she does... but with a lot of vaginal pain, even worse than before. The sex therapist, secretly feeling defeated, refers Marcia to a well-known urogynecologist for a "second" (which is actually now the 4th healthcare provider) opinion. Then come the tissue biopsies, more laparoscopic "exploratory" surgeries and nerve blocks. Marcia's physical, mental and emotional health starts to take a downward spiral out of control. She is now a 26yr old, nearly divorced, depressed female who can't sit in a chair for more than 30 minutes due to constant, severe pelvic pain.

Sound unbelievable? Well, believe it! As mentioned above, I see at least one new "Marcia" every week with a similar story of multiple treatments and surgeries by several, highly educated and well trained healthcare professionals but without getting relief. How could such competent doctors seem so clueless when it comes to a problem such as Marcia's? Perhaps the problem is due to seeking out help from the wrong specialty. The only healthcare profession that looks at muscles as the **source** of pain is physical therapy and this profession is not historically known as first responders for problems such as pelvic pain or pain with intercourse.

Think about this. There are physicians for nerves, physicians for bones, physicians for the heart and lungs, blood vessels, endocrine system, gastrointestinal tract, kidneys, bladder, reproductive system, skin, internal medicine, but there are NO physicians strictly for muscles. But most people don't know that. Therefore, they go to a seemingly related physician for a problem that may be originating within the pelvic floor muscles, (an area that the majority of doctors are not experts in), and expect them to give the magic "pill" *(or at least the answer to the problem)*.

The second concern is most healthcare professionals are attempting to successfully treat a single problem that is clearly multifaceted. When a woman has pain in an area of her body that defines her femininity, it affects her physical body as well as her thoughts, emotions and her sense of well-being…her sense of self. Not to mention, the damage that *chronic* pain has on a family structure. The lack of intimacy with her spouse, the increased responsibility on family members for emotional and physical support and, sometimes, role reversals regarding care-giving within the home. These changes can be particularly damaging to the family unit. As seen in Marcia's case, if physician #1 or even #2 had pulled in help from a sex therapist and a pelvic floor specialist, perhaps Marcia's condition would not have progressed and intensified as it did. Perhaps Marcia's mental state and sense of self could have been preserved early on. Please don't misunderstand, physicians *are just as* important as pelvic floor therapists and psychologists when it comes to creating a plan of care for patients with pelvic pain and painful intercourse.

As a pelvic floor specialist, I prefer patients to be managed medically, either hormonally and/or with analgesics, so I can perform the necessary treatments directly to the affected pelvic floor tissues. If the patient is too sensitive to touch, then evaluation and treatment will be difficult to carry out. Additionally, hormonal regulation and/or maintenance are also critical pieces of the pelvic pain puzzle. Hormones help create a vaginal environment where the tissues are well lubricated and resistant to micro-tearing or friction injuries. Also, hormones are key to bulking up pelvic floor muscles to allow and improve the quality of contraction and ability for muscle contraction AND relaxation.

Additionally, and of equal importance is managing the mental and emotional well-being of the patient with appropriate counseling. Since I am not a psychologist, I am not at liberty, or trained to discuss formal psychological treatment protocols for women, and men, affected by sexual dysfunctions and pain. However, I will concede this important factor. In a perfect world, all three treatment plans provided by the physician, the pelvic specialist and psychologist would operate in chorus with one another to bring healing and restoration to the individual as a whole. Members of each discipline, skilled and competent in their own expertise, would work in unity with each other by means of open communication, sharing their ideas and knowledge, and operating fully within their specialty to deliver cutting edge treatments. Patients would receive a customized plan of care to meet their needs and established goals. It's a win/win for everyone. The healthcare providers feel a sense of gratitude and accomplishment that they are providing the best care for their patient and the patient is the recipient of healing. A treatment plan like this sets the patient up for the best results and brings long-lasting relief.

Now let's assume you're under appropriate medical and psychological management for painful intercourse. What is a pelvic floor specialist and what can they do? A pelvic floor specialist is a women's health physical therapist who has gone through extensive training and/or rigorous testing and who has substantial hours of clinical, hands-on experience dealing with patients suffering with pelvic floor dysfunctions/disorders, including pelvic pain. Pelvic floor specialists are considered experts in pelvic floor anatomy and should be able to easily identify and care for problems related to the pelvic floor. Pelvic floor specialists treat individuals with a variety of diagnoses including, but not limited to, vulvodynia, vaginismus, vestibulodynia, coccydynia, constipation, interstitial cystitis, urinary or fecal incontinence, overactive bladder, organ prolapse, and dyspareunia/pain during intercourse. There are many variations of techniques that these specialists might use on their patients. I will discuss several techniques I use and find most beneficial in my clinic.

So, what specific pelvic floor rehabilitation treatments are available for pain during intercourse? Before deciding on the best plan of care, it's essential to step back and take a look at the entire picture. I first gather information regarding a patient's medical history, old injuries, current pain levels, diet, hygiene, typical daily tasks, career duties and/or family/spousal support. During this interview, I will also inquire about when they experience their pain and if it's position dependent or cyclic. If I see areas of concern, I will make specific suggestions regarding diet modifications, body mechanics training and postural education. If needed, I will also suggest referrals to other healthcare professionals where appropriate. For instance, if the patient indicates that they have cyclic pain or are experiencing hormonal changes, such as hot flashes, weight fluctuations, low libido, hair loss, etc. I would most likely refer the patient to a gynecologist.

Once a good history is obtained, a thorough external and internal evaluation is performed to identify the dysfunctions. Starting broad, posture and body movements are observed and accessory muscles to the pelvic floor are carefully assessed to determine if muscular trigger points, myofascial restrictions and movement dysfunctions are present. Many times, these seemingly unrelated restrictions contribute significantly to pain during intercourse and should not be overlooked. Often, if these areas are ignored, pelvic pain may not be fully resolved and/or become a recurrent problem. After getting a general impression of the overall body, it's time to narrow things down to the pelvic exam.

Women who have had significant discomfort going to a gynecologist may become apprehensive with the idea of having an internal vaginal examination; However, let me put the brain at ease and say there are no stirrups or speculum used when performing this kind of evaluation *(Thank God for that!)*. Thus, toleration during this kind of examination is typically easier to handle and less intimidating.

Through the vaginal canal, the pelvic floor muscles can be thoroughly assessed and treated. Manual techniques, such as trigger point release, myofascial release, scar mobilization, stretching, manual biofeedback, soft tissue mobility and neural glides, can be performed directly to pelvic floor muscles, nerves and surrounding tissues….and with great success, I might add! Other common manual techniques including fascial manipulation, intramuscular trigger point release (also known as dry needling), strain/counter-strain, pelvic and sacral mobilizations are also very helpful techniques for alleviating pelvic pain symptoms.

In my opinion, manual therapy is a necessity for resolving pelvic pain and pain during intercourse and is often the missing link amongst healthcare providers' treatment plans. Although these manual techniques are considered the foundation of pelvic rehabilitation, they are not the only effective treatments. Other important strategies for healing pelvic floor and vaginal pain during intercourse include education and training regarding motor (muscle) control, down-training spastic or tight muscles, diet modifications, body mechanics and/or postural adjustments, physiological quieting, stretches (legs, hips and pelvic floor via dilation). Although these techniques don't seem impressive, they are vital for achieving lasting results as well as managing chronic conditions independently. What good is manually relaxing a muscle if you can't teach the recipient how to maintain that relaxation at home?

Part 2: Staying Connected With Intimacy

Although there are a variety of treatments that are available and quite successful for women with painful intercourse, some individuals have multiple health conditions or complications that hinder intimacy on a regular basis. What about these ladies? How can they maintain a sexual closeness with their spouse that is also gratifying for them?

Many individuals find it difficult to be intimate with their mates when they are dealing with chronic health conditions because they don't know what to do and/or how much to do without flaring up their symptoms. Often they operate in fear when it comes to sexual intimacy and resist the idea of trying anything new. Eventually, guilt about not pleasuring her man sets in and sexual tension between the couple peaks, resulting in a very guarded wife "giving in" to her husband for the night. Afterwards, she's confirmed that she doesn't like sex nor does she want to try it anytime soon and he feels rejected and bad about causing his wife's symptoms to increase. Obviously, not an ideal situation.

Chronic conditions and health problems makes intimacy a bit more complicated but certainly not impossible. First, be clear about what you are willing or not willing to try prior to climbing under the sheets. For example, if you have a bladder condition, such as interstitial cystitis, then spend as little time as possible touching or applying direct pressure over the bladder or urethra. When talking it through with your spouse, encourage and show him where it's okay to touch and teach him how you'd like to be stimulated. With painful conditions of the bladder and/or vaginal canal, perform lots of foreplay and keep the penile thrusting to a minimum. In other words, stimulate your husband to a heightened state, waiting to the very end to enter the vagina prior to climax. Keep the thrusting to two to four pumps at the most. This is a helpful tip for anyone with trouble tolerating penile thrusting.

Performing "outer-course" can be as enjoyable as intercourse. Outer-course is sexual touching, kissing, caressing, cuddling, licking, tickling, nibbling and/or stroking everywhere but inside. It's known as non-penetrative sex. It's very powerful and often can bring both partners to orgasmic ecstasy. Maybe your outer-course includes rubbing or massaging the vulva, stimulating the clitoris or performing oral sex. It's whatever you and your spouse are comfortable with. Be sure to incorporate the penis in your foreplay and/or outer-course so that he still feels engaged and connected throughout your entire love-making session.

With chronic conditions, take advantage of your "good days". If you are feeling good, plant a love seed for your husband through a note inviting him to perform certain acts with you at a specified time of day. By the way, it's helpful if you plan for a time that you'll be alert and awake! Don't be afraid to ask your physician for medications that may help you enjoy or tolerate sexual intercourse, such as lidocaine. If you take medications for your chronic condition, be sure not to skip taking the medication on the day you're planning to be intimate. In addition to taking your medications, prepare your body with relaxation methods, down-training techniques and/or stretching exercises prior to getting under the sheets. Take a warm shower or bath, if needed, to help relax your muscles and your mind. Try stretching and/or restorative yoga to help further relax your muscles. Planning ahead will give you a sense of control and a better outcome overall. Once you find and establish ways to enjoy sex with your husband without flaring your condition, sex will be more enjoyable and perhaps more frequent.

CHAPTER EIGHT

I like it like that!
Orthopedic Considerations for Intimacy

"Sex is only painful when he puts this leg up by my shoulder and around my head while pushing this leg to the other side," says a former patient of mine as she demonstrates the fully clothed version of her sex position in the waiting room chair. As I stood amazed how anyone could want or enjoy sex in that position, I began wrestling with the reason why couples seek out and try crazy sex positions during intercourse. What are the benefits for having her legs up by her ears? What are the potential dangers? Where are her "hot spots" located when trying these positions and/or are they even accessible? What about chronic conditions such as back pain or bladder pain? Are these positions better or worse for those types of disorders? These questions sparked enough inside of me to turn on my "research mode".

There are several things one must consider when choosing the right position for intimacy. First and foremost, what is the goal? Do you want to maintain stimulation and arousal during penile thrusting? Do you want to climax at the same time as your spouse? Are you focusing on relaxation of the pelvic floor muscles? Are you trying to achieve a tighter fit around the penis? Or are you just bored with "getting it on" in the same position? What is the number one goal that you are trying to attain during your sexual encounter?

Your goals do not have to be set in stone, either. In fact, your goals may change with every love encounter or perhaps, if the love-making session is particularly lengthy, within the same session. Some days, your goal may be to maintain sexual arousal and stimulation throughout the entire love making process with the intention of coming to a beautiful, intense climatic ending in unison with your mate. Whereas other days, time may be of essence for you and therefore, your goal may be to jump on the fast track and have a "quickie," if you will. For some individuals, the goal may always be to avoid painful or uncomfortable areas as well as reduce the risks of potential flares ups in pain, as seen in many chronic pain conditions. Whatever the reason, understanding your goal *AND* communicating it to your spouse is essential when agreeing to perform in certain sexual positions.

Let's consider several potential goals that many individuals actively seek out when having sex. This will not be an all-inclusive descriptive list, rather it's meant to be viewed as a general guideline offering choices to help you achieve your intimacy goals. Creativity and human anatomy truly dictates what works best for couples. Some couples may find that the "basics" work quite well for them whereas others may need ideas for improved connectivity and pleasure. Regardless of where you are in your relationship, here are some suggestions to improve comfort and excitement, create newness, and/or increase sexual arousal/sensation.

The first, most obvious and most common, goal for couples is to increase sensation or arousal with the hope to reach orgasm.

For women, it is essential to know and understand your body's response to touch. What feels good to you? What feels bad or annoying to you? You may need to take one entire love-making session just to figure that out. As mentioned above, try using your husband's penis to stimulate various areas of your vulva and/or vagina to help confirm your favorite pleasure zones. Once you find these areas, you can plan ahead the positions you'd like to try at the next encounter.

Let's say you are like 90% of women in this country and prefer clitoral stimulation. Then, it's fair to say, you should choose positions that allow easy access to the clitoris. The easiest of positions for direct clitoral stimulation include face to face, female on her back with her legs opened and clitoris exposed. This is known as the missionary position. Her knees are typically bent up, supported by pillows or wrapped around her mate. This is a position that will definitely unveil the delicate structure of the clitoris so be sure to educate your spouse on how to proceed when he gets here (i.e. how much pressure he should apply, speed of stimulation, location of stimulation, etc.). If the clitoris is erect and the tissues have pulled away, sometimes pressure from the male pubic bone creates enough stimulation during penile thrusting to produce sustained arousal or orgasm.

In this missionary position, the breasts are also exposed and can easily be caressed, with or without nipple stimulation (again, based on personal preference). Remember, there are some women who can reach orgasm with nipple stimulation alone, and a whole lot more of us that need other areas stimulated before that can happen. For these breast-stimulated women, if sexual arousal is a primary goal, then face to face positions may offer pleasurable benefits during *every* sexual encounter. The missionary position can also give way to manual or penile stimulation to the G-spot or the A-spot (if you so desire).

Face to face love-making can also allow for kissing, groping and caressing the breast, thighs, locking fingers with your partner, reading their facial expressions (determining delight or pain) and it also allows for control of penile thrusting speed and depth. If he is on top, he is able to penetrate deeply into the vaginal canal and at the desirable speed. If she is on top, she can control how deeply he enters and, again, the speed at which she prefers it to happen. This is ideal for a woman who may not enjoy or tolerate full penetration from her spouse or who needs a very slow entry. Depth should not be too much of a concern for men as the majority of their sexual sensation comes from the first 1 ½ to 2 inches of the tip of their penis.

Face to face love-making does not refer to missionary style exclusively. There are many variations to this that are helpful for producing pleasure. Face to face positions can also include her straddling him while he is lying on his back OR both partners lying on their sides with her top leg draped over his hip OR her sitting on his lap while he embraces her body close to his. Be as creative as you'd like with these face to face love-making positions, coming into and out of these variations as comfort and time allows. However, remember a few key things. The closer your knees and legs are to your chest, the deeper the penile penetration, perhaps increased stimulation to G or A spots (if that is one of your arousing zones), but the less control you have and decreased ability for clitoral stimulation. The lower your knees/legs, the more pelvic floor relaxation, improved control over depth and/or speed of penetration, improved clitoral stimulation and accessibility to the breasts for caressing or stimulation. Due to being able to stimulate several arousing areas, face to face positions may be the best for increasing the potential of multiple orgasms with little interruption.

What if your goal is to make a tighter fit around your husband?... *increase the friction, if you will.* The position of intimacy that may work best for you would be rear entry….not to be confused with rectal entry. With rear entry positions, the man would enter the vaginal canal from behind as opposed to the front. In this position, the pelvic floor muscles have more tension and therefore, there is a tighter squeeze around the penis upon entry and thrusting. The rear entry sex position that I am referring to is known to the general public as "doggy style", which for most women, the name alone is a huge turn-off. Let's call this position "quadruped style" instead. Essentially, the woman is on her hands and knees and her man is entering from behind. In the quadruped position, the man can reach around to provide clitoral stimulation; however, it may be a difficult task to perform due to lack of visualization or simply due to his arm's length. The quadruped position does not offer a lot of control for the female, but will produce a snugger fit for both.

Other rear entry positions include the woman lying completely flat on her stomach and the man supporting himself with his arms with penile entry from behind or both partners can be lying on their side woman in front of her mate (in the spoon position). Some women find rear entry less intimidating if they are lying on their stomachs or on their sides versus the quadruped position. Also, with these latter positions, depth of penetration is slightly hindered by her buttocks and therefore, tends to be more comfortable for women who have trouble tolerating deep penetration.

Comfort is an important component of enjoying sex and wanting to have more of it. Finding positions of comfort, such as in the rear entry "spooning" position, is unique to the physical anatomy that is involved. What I mean is you must always consider the male anatomy. Is he curved a little to the left or right? Is he slightly tilted down or is he standing straight up? Considering the male anatomy is just as important as knowing your own hot spots and what turns you on. There are plenty of men that have mild curves to their penis during erections. Most of the time, these curves go unnoticed by their female partners. However, in some cases, if the female is experiencing some kind of pelvic problem, (i.e. bladder or urethral pain, rectal pain/pressure, hip pain, pulled groin, organ prolapse, etc.), then she will need to consider her spouse's anatomy when choosing a comfortable sex position.

Imagine with me, a banana. Be sure you're imaging a long banana with a slight curve and not one of those small, curled up dwarf bananas. Now, if your husband is slightly curved up (tip the banana upwards in your mind), then every time you try sex in the missionary position, his penis will bump into the bladder during each thrust, particularly deep thrusting. If your bladder and urethra are irritated after sex or you have an existing bladder condition (I.C., overactive bladder or bladder prolapse), you may want to choose a rear entry positions to avoid or limit contact with the bladder. Now, turn your banana to the side a little. If your husband is curved slightly to the side, right or left, and you have hip pain or low back pain; you may want to choose a sex position that avoids pressure against the side that hurts. The same applies for symptoms of rectal pressure, chronic constipation or pain. Again, the point is, you must consider the male anatomy to improve your comfort. You can use this same strategy for helping improve stimulation to your inner erogenous zones. So, if you like G-spot stimulation, you may want your curved penis to touch that with every thrust to improve your chances of having an orgasm at the same time.

What do you like? What do you want out of your sexual relationship? Ask yourself these questions and make the answers known to your partner….clearly known. Remember, if he knew, he would have done it by now, so don't force him to guess. Spell it out, act it out, write it out, diagram it if you need. Make it easy for him. If you simply don't know, then try something new with him. Just because you didn't like something (e.g. breast stimulation) one day, doesn't mean you won't like it another day. As mentioned before, hormones can play a major role in stimulation and arousal based on the time of the month. Keep your mind opened and together you will come up with positions that you both love.

CHAPTER NINE

Dead in the Bed?
Get Your Groove Back!

Ask any person under the age of 40 years what sex will be like when they are in their 70's and they usually laugh out loud, alluding to the idea of non-existent. It's tempting to think that as we age, we stop being sexual or sexually stimulated. The truth be told, it's not age that stops us from making love. In fact, there are countless polls out there that report statistics contrary to the elderly celibate vow. Curiosity has led many researchers to conduct polls concluding that the elderly are still quite sexually active. One supportive study published by About.com, from Dr. Mark Stibich, found that out of 3,000 people polled, 70% of individuals in their late 50s/early 60s, 53% of those aged 65-74 and 26% of individuals 75 or older are still getting it on (*Hey, in the 75 year and older category, that's 1 in 4 people!*). Of course, Viagra helps these statistics a little bit! But whatever you gotta do to get the job done, do it! The primary reason these percentages decline with age is because one half of the couple usually dies and the social network of the surviving partner is typically minimal to choose from.

So, if it isn't age, what makes couples sexually dead in the bed? Sex and marriage psychologist/counselors agree that sexless marriages start out like most, full of love, passion, respect, excitement and, well, lots of sex. However, as time passes, daily stresses and lack of communication start to wedge their way between the loving couple. The couple starts to build up resentment and/or anger towards each other. They stop trying to woo each other or show their appreciation for their better halves. Sex becomes more like a chore, boring or uneventful and, as time wanes on, less frequent or extinct even. Perhaps, his/her physical appearance starts to decline intermingled with feelings of no longer being desirable. Eventually, these thoughts start manifesting into explosive conflicts over who took the dog out last or who will clean the dishes. Combine this scenario with hormone imbalances and/or low libido and you get a perfect recipe for divorce....or at least the fantasy of one.

So is there hope for unhappy, sexless married couples? Of course there is! Otherwise, there would be no point to writing this book! There is always hope for those who seek it! If this is you and I've just described your marriage, the question you should ask yourself is, "Do I want better?" A better point of view. A better relationship. A better sex life. The mere fact that you are reading this book says YES, you do. Having a better sex life is just a portion of restoring a healthy marriage, but a big portion at that. So, where do you start?

Since the majority of your sexual arousal and experience begins in your brain, let's start there. We discussed confirmation bias in a previous chapter and the dangers of allowing yourself to think and confirm negative thoughts about your spouse. Well, you can use this same principle for positive confirmation. Try thinking something positive about your spouse. (For some of you, this may be difficult, but not impossible). Maybe you say to yourself, "(Insert husband's name) is a hard worker." Then, you begin to confirm that thought. "See how he is taking the trash out without me even asking". "Look at how he puts the dishes in the sink (they may not make it to the dishwasher, but be optimistic)." "I really appreciate him getting the children ready for bed tonight." Use as many positive examples to affirm your thought(s) about him. Every time you think of something negative about your spouse, try replacing it with something positive about him. Eventually, you'll start thinking more optimistically about your relationship overall.

Once you start changing your thought process, find activities or interests you can share or do together with your spouse. If it's eating, try a new restaurant, cook together or go grocery shopping at an exotic food market. Maybe, if you are feeling down about your appearance, you start an exercise program with your husband. Perhaps you set time to take a walk every evening together or plan weekend biking or hiking trips. Try setting a date night every week that you are committing exclusively for each other. Perhaps you play a game or cuddle on the couch to watch a movie. It really doesn't matter as long as you are spending time with each other. Can't think of something? Do a Google search on the internet. There are a million suggestions with countless possibilities! Pick one and commit to it each week.

It's ironic how the person you couldn't stop thinking about, touching and talking to at one point in your life is the same person with whom you have trouble communicating today… *and after all these years*. However, every expert across America would agree that communication is the key to a good relationship and a necessary component to great sex. Sometimes individuals experience new dysfunctions that are difficult to talk about with their spouse, such as pelvic pain, vaginal dryness or anorgasmia (inability to have an orgasm). For men, perhaps he has developed erectile dysfunction or premature ejaculation, something he may have never experienced before. Whatever the problem, communicate with your spouse about the sexual dysfunctions or sexual frustrations and know that, 9 times out of 10, there is help available. Discuss your options and allow your mate to offer support. Don't be afraid to admit to your troubles with low libido or poor stimulation. It might be something he is experiencing too. We have already discussed how common low libido is for women and the role hormones play. However, hormonal imbalances don't just affect women, but men, as well, particularly as they age. If your man is always tired, gaining weight, feeling depressed, has low libido, losing his hair, etc., chances are he has low testosterone. A simple blood test and testosterone medication or supplements is all it takes sometimes to make a Rambo (or a Brad Pitt…a Denzel Washington…a Ryan Gosling…a Mario Lopez…) out of your man.

Some of you are LOL-ing right now because you are saying to yourself, "Have you seen my husband?" There is no way we're making a Denzel out of him! You are missing the point! The point is, when you and he start feeling better about yourselves and each other, then sex becomes exciting again. Sex should be fun not boring. Too many people describe their sex lives as an obligatory act rather than a fun experience. Several patients have shared similar stories regarding their sex lives sounding something like this:

> He says he wants to have sex. It seems like he ***always*** wants to have sex. I can't keep holding him off, or shouldn't, so I finally agree. I lay there and wait for him to be finished and then we go to bed.

Perhaps the deadness in the bed is because sex isn't fun anymore. Where is the laughter and the horseplay? What happened to the gentle teasing and banter you did when you were first in love? It's okay to have serious sex every once and in a while, but playful sex is really enjoyable too! Sometimes, particularly if you've been with each other for a long time, you fall into a routine of "this is the way we do it" and you get stuck there. You stop trying to make each other smile. You stop flirting and settle for the "same ol', same ol'." Try changing up your sexual positions or the places you have sex. Don't always expect your husband to be the master mind of all things sexual. Try planning ahead and create a bedroom scene of sensual bliss that captivates your 5 senses (as discussed earlier). Be creative and take your husband off guard every now and then. Having trouble coming up with something romantic? One word…Pinterest.

Being creative is a great way to restore romance in your marriage. It helps you to step out of your complacency and communicates to your spouse that "Hey, I've been intentionally thinking of you and went out of my way to show you that I want you sexually." Men love that! But even creativity, at times, has a hard time competing with a women's multi-tasking brain. It's difficult to stop our brains from thinking of more than just one thing at a time. We may start off enjoying the moment, but if left untamed, the brain will begin to drift off to other tasks and

To-Do's of the day…or the following day (depending on when you're getting it on). How can romance compete with that?

Multi-tasking while making love is a great way to kill romance **unless** you are using it to your advantage. *Say WHAT?!?* You can condition your brain to multitask in such a way that it enhances your sexual experience. Women with heightened sexual arousal, who have no trouble with libido, do all the time do this. We talked about this earlier, but try fantasizing about your lover and your love making experience. Think about how you and he are connecting during intercourse and break it down as if you were reading your very own love novel. Describe, in your mind, how he is kissing your lips or neck and how he is caressing your breast or running his fingertips down your back. Then confirm to yourself how that is making you feel. Hopefully, you are using positive confirmation! If not, you **must** communicate those things that annoy you to your spouse and give him the opportunity to correct himself. Again, make your love novel as graphic and as detailed as you wish. Keep your mind engaged in your novel as the love-making plays out. As you start to feel stimulated and aroused, tell yourself how good that makes you feel. Confirm how you love feeling sexually stimulated and allow yourself to be overwhelmed with sexy thoughts about your husband and what he is doing to you. If you've never done this, it may feel a little awkward at first, but the more you keep your brain and body engaged, the more you will enjoy the experience. Practicing fantasy like this will help you stay focused on the moment and, in turn, keep the arousal heightened. It will also help with building anticipation about your next love encounter!

Whether your marriage's sexiness has died with age or has become boring and uneventful, know that it can be resurrected with a little effort and experimentation. This is certainly not a one way street rather a journey for you and your spouse to explore. Both can practice positive confirmation. Both can make intentional efforts to be involved in regular communication and quality time. And, although men do not need this as much, both can be involved in sexual fantasy about their mates. It truly is a win-win for your marriage!

CHAPTER TEN

Striving for Better

Sex with your soul mate is a beautiful act. It was never designed for a 50% success rate. That is, only one of the two individuals achieving sexual gratification or climax. Rather, it was divinely designed so that a man and woman could become one in their mind, body and spirit (i.e. complete sexual satisfaction). Throughout the years, corruption and media fabrications have tainted the beauty of sex and turned it into unrealistic ideations of how two people exchange intimacy. As a result, many men and women are sent confusing signals and/or images about their role in intercourse. The resulting factor is the resounding 80% of women who do not reach climax or sexual fulfillment during intimacy.

Admittedly, we women are often difficult to figure out sexually. Sometimes we want it this way and other times we don't. Our indecisiveness is driven by hormonal cycles, at times, poor knowledge about what structures are made for stimulation and how our bodies respond uniquely from our counterpart. Even taking care of our bodies has been a challenge because it's not common knowledge and rarely discussed with healthcare providers. I mean, who knew you were never supposed to use soap "down there" or that certain lubrications could increase your risk for infections. One thing you can be sure of is the majority of women desire to be sexually satisfied. Sometimes they just don't know how to get there.

Women have historically taken a backseat to initiating or being an active participate in sexual intercourse. They expect to operate primarily as the receiver and rarely as the giver which can be very frustrating to men, at times. Poor knowledge about how to reach sexual climax aids in the passivity of women because neither partner knows what's involved to achieve an orgasm for her. She is often left feeling that sex is not a big deal and not worth the effort. Until now!

Women have a greater role in sex than once thought or accepted. She has the power to improve her sexual experience through discovering her hot spots, guiding her partner with direction on how to stimulate and taking responsibility for her own libido. Although low libido is common, it's not normal and, best of all, it can be helped. In fact, many sexual dysfunctions can be successfully treated with a skilled team of healthcare providers who are familiar and experienced with pelvic floor conditions. Sometimes, simple, non-medical changes in behavior and preparations can really affect how she approaches sex and how she responds. It's a matter of striving for better in your intimate relationship. Ladies, if you are unhappy with your current sex life, take this knowledge and run!

Don't get locked into thinking that the sex positions you liked at age 25 should be sufficient or as good at age 55. Your body changes and, trust me; things are not in the same position as they once were! Try new positions, particularly if you are dealing with chronic conditions or injuries such as low back or hip pain. Keep trying new areas to stimulate and/or arouse periodically.

Hormonal changes throughout the month, and even as we age, can dictate what feels good one day and awful on another day. So, don't be too quick to give up.

Reading What a Girl Wants is just the first step to a happier sex life. It's up to you to take the information and apply it to your marriage. Have your husband read it or educate him so he can have a deeper understanding and compassion about how your body operates. Sex is a bit like coffee. If you've had a lot of it over the years, it doesn't seem to have the same exhilarating effects on your body as it did in the beginning...***unless*** you hit it with a flavor shot.

CHAPTER ELEVEN

FAQ's
Real Questions from Real Women

- What is considered a "good" sex life? How many times a week or month should a couple be having sex?
  - o Frequency of intercourse is very couple-specific. A good sex life can be once a week to everyday of the week. It is dependent on work schedules, travel schedules, illnesses, time constraints, etc. A "sexless marriage" by definition is being sexually intimate less than 10 times per year. That's close to 1x/month. Therefore, a healthy sex life would be *at least* once per month. Discuss this topic with your spouse and come to an agreement on your frequency of intimacy. Give yourselves a goal to strive for every month. The more positive experiences you have with intimacy, the increased likelihood that you'll desire to do it again and again.

- Certain times of the month, it feels like my husband is hitting the back of my vagina. What is that?

- Just after ovulation and during menses, the cervix drops 2-4cm towards the vaginal opening. If you feel the symptoms only when you are engaging in intercourse during these times of the month, he is most likely hitting your cervix with deep penile thrusting.
- There is another situation that can provoke the sensation of "hitting a wall" and that is from severe muscle tension. If the pelvic floor muscles are tight and spastic, the penis will have trouble entering the vaginal canal, if at all. If this is your situation, please know there is help. These muscles can be released and relaxed with a specialist trained in pelvic floor rehabilitation.

- Will using a vibrator all the time hurt my vagina?
  - No, it will not "hurt" your vagina, but it may make it difficult for your husband to bring you to orgasm without it. Also, over time, your tissues may become desensitized which could temporarily cause anorgasmia (inability to achieve an orgasm). Don't worry! If you give the vibrator a break, this should resolve over a period of time and you'll be able to reach orgasm once again.

- How can I have more than one orgasm during intercourse?
  - As mentioned above, having multiple orgasms is easier for women than men due to a shorter refractory (recovery) period after the first orgasm. Sometimes, continued stimulation to the same arousal zone could produce an immediate peak and a second orgasm. However, this area may become extremely sensitive or

even painful after the initial orgasm. If so, a separate arousal area must be stimulated in order to have a second orgasm. Try both ways to see what will work best for you. Remember, there are many areas on a woman's body that can bring her to orgasm. Knowing the location of these areas is half the battle!

- Will using olive oil decrease the effectiveness of a condom?
    o Yes, olive oil (and other oil or petroleum based lubricants) has the potential to break down condoms hence lose its purpose. The best type of lubricant to use with condoms is water-based, glycerin-free lubricants. Do a quick internet search with the key words "Water Based Personal Lubricants" and you'll find several options that will work great with condoms.

- Does size really matter?
    o In general, size does not matter. The average erect male penis in the United States is approximately 5 inches in length and 4-5 inches in diameter. Believe it or not, other countries have different averages for the adult erect male penis. For the purpose of this book, we are going with the United States' norms. Since, the average vagina is 4-6 inches in depth and 2 inches in width, at rest, and the vaginal tissues are able to stretch beyond your wildest imagination, it is accommodating to most any size penis. I often remind my patients, if a baby's head can come out, a penis can surely go in. Women have the most vaginal sensitivity 1-2 inches inside the vaginal opening whereas men have the most sensitivity

1-2 inches from the tip of their penis. So, if you're married to a man that is a little on the smaller size, it won't make a difference to you or him! Remember, it's not the size of the boat, but the motion of the ocean!

- Sometimes after sex, I have a little blood. Is that normal?
  o Post-coital bleeding is not normal and should be addressed. Bleeding occurs when the vaginal tissues become dry and fragile and/or the muscles have atrophied (i.e. wasted away). The bleeding is a result of a friction injury from the penis moving back/forth. This is a common finding in women that are menopausal, but can also happen to younger women on birth control pills. Hormones are to blame in both cases. Menopausal women should ask their gynecologist about vaginal hormones to help bulk up the tissues and muscles as well as keep them well lubricated. For the younger women on birth control pills, there are many pills or alternatives out on the market that may work best for you. Discuss your symptoms of vaginal dryness with your physician to determine what option is best for you. For women with vaginal dryness, foreplay and lots of lubrication is a must!

- Sometimes when I'm having sex, I start out aroused, but then I quickly lose interest. Is there something wrong with me?
  o This is a very common problem for many women. The two main culprits are lack of continued stimulation to your hot spots AND a multi-tasking brain at work. Educated your mate on all the places you love touched,

kissed, nibbled and teased and keep your brain engaged with his play-by-play moves on your body!

- I feel like I smell "down there." I don't have any weird discharge or pain, just a strong odor. Is that normal?
    o Vaginal odors are the resultant of several factors. Most odors are completely normal and a result of hormones and/or hormonal changes/imbalances. The ironic thing about vaginal odors is that you are most likely the only one who picks up on it. Most men are not aware of vaginal odors or find it very appealing. Often, it is what drives him to you! Odors can also be caused by diet. Some foods cause a strange, or more intense, odor in your urine and/or vagina. Example foods include coffee, garlic, onions, asparagus, excessive meat, dairy or alcohol. Try modifying your diet to see if the odor changes.
    o Odor that is foul-smelling, different from your "normal", and is typically accompanied by green, yellow or white-clumpy discharge is indicative of some kind of infection. This may or may not be painful or with/without a fever. This requires medical management or intervention and should be addressed by your gynecologist.

- Sometimes after having sex with my husband, I pass gas out of my vagina. Should I be worried?
    o Believe it or not, there is a term for this. It's called vaginal flatulence. It may occur during and/or after intercourse and is the result of air being trapped

inside the vagina canal. Certain sexual positions and/or vaginal dryness will increase the likelihood of vaginal flatulence. Typically, there is not a foul odor when it happens; however, should a foul odor or fecal matter accompany the vaginal flatulence, seek medical attention immediately. It is a sign of something more series and/or life-threatening.

- o Sometimes air is getting trapped inside the vagina because there is little support and/or stability around the vaginal canal. In other words, your muscles have become weakened causing the vagina to be more opened and loose. Pelvic floor muscle exercises and core stabilization are perfect solutions for this type of problem and should do the trick to resolve these unwanted sounds.

- I have had three babies and, as a result, my vagina feels like a big, open cave? What can I do to make my vagina tighter?
    - o Children are a joy and a blessing, but they really can change a woman's body significantly. It is common to have pelvic floor muscle weakness after having one or more vaginal births. The good news is, just like your arm or leg muscles, the pelvic floor muscles can be strengthened. Stronger muscles make for a tighter fit for you and him. These muscles, most likely, will not be as they were before you started having children, but with a little training and consistency they will be significantly improved.

- I can't have an orgasm during intercourse. My husband has been with other women before me and he seems surprised that I can't orgasm with just in and out thrusting. Am I the only one with this problem?
    - No. In fact, you are "normal." The majority of women, 75-80%, cannot have an orgasm with in and out thrusting alone. They require clitoral stimulation or stimulation to an arousal zone. Which means, many women have lied (eh hum…faked it) about having orgasm during intercourse.

- How long should sex last?
    - Sexual intimacy is made up of kissing, foreplay, intercourse, post-intercourse cuddling, etc. and can take minutes to hours depending on the couple and the amount of time they have devoted to love-making. Actual intercourse (in/out thrusting) typically lasts about 8-12 minutes, give or take a minute. Men that ejaculate after 2-3 minutes of stimulation are said to have premature ejaculation. However, if you are performing external stimulation to him prior to insertion, then that counts towards the "2-3 minutes rule" and he may actually be able to last much longer. Some women, like those with pelvic pain, may purposefully try to stimulate their men externally to keep the time inside the vagina to a minimal. If you count the time of kissing, foreplay, intercourse and post cuddling, then the entire process may take 30-60 minutes. The most important part of sex is not the time it takes, but the enjoyment of the process.

REFERENCES

1) Abramov L A. Sexual life and frigidity among women developing acute myocardial infarction. *Psychosom Med.* 1976;38:418-25.
2) Butler S M, Snowdon D A. Trends in mortality in older women: findings from the nun study. *J Gerontol Ser B.* 1996;51:S201-8.
3) Choi, Charles. February 23, 2013. *A Curvy body's like a drug to men*.nbcnews.com/health. Retrieved from http://www.nbcnews.com/id/35540957/ns/health-skin_and_beauty/t/curvy-bodys-drug-men/#.UgESQZKkqJl.
4) Davey Smith, G., Frankel S., Yarnell, J. *Sex and Death: are they related? Findings from the Caerphilly Cohort Study.* BMJ 1997 Dec 20-27;315(7123): 1641-4.
5) Donaldson James, S. September 4, 2009. *Female Orgasm May Be Tied to 'Rule of Thumb'.* ABCNEWS.com/health. Retrieved from http://abcnews.go.com/Health/ReproductiveHealth/sex-study-female-orgasm-eludes-majority-women/story?id=8485289&page=2#.T5vI6KsV3fY
6) Goldstein, A., Brandon, M. *Reclaiming Desire: 4 Keys to Finding Your Lost Libido.* Rodale.
7) Herrera, I. (2009). *Ending female pain: A woman's manual.* Duplex Publishing.
8) Herrera, I. June 26, 2012. *Overcoming Pelvic Pain: When treating pelvic dysfunction, not all Kegels are created equal.* Advance for

    <u>Physical Therapy and Rehab Medicine. Retrieved from http://physical-therapy.advanceweb.com/Features/Articles/Overcoming-Pelvic-Pain.aspx</u>

9) Joseph A. Flaherty, John Marcell Davis, Philip G. Janicak (1993, Digitized Oct 29, 2010). *Psychiatry: Diagnosis & therapy. A Lange clinical manual*. Appleton & Lange (Original from Northwestern University). pp. 544 pages. <u>ISBN</u> <u>0-8385-1267-4, 9780838512678</u>. Retrieved January 5, 2012.

10) Kaplan S D. Retrospective cohort mortality study of Roman Catholic priests. *Prev Med*. 1988;17:335-343.

11) Levin R, and Meston C. Nipple/breast stimulation and sexual arousal in young men and women. J Sex Med 2006;3:450–454.

12) Masters & Johnson *Human Sexual Response,* Bantam, 1981 ISBN 978-055-3204292; 1st ed. 1966.

13) Masters, William H., Virginia E., Johnson, Reproductive Biology Research Foundation (U.S.) 1966. *Human Sexual Response*. Little, Brown, p.366. ISBN 0-316-54987-8.9780316549875.

14) <u>McAnulty, R.D., Burnette, M.M. *Sexuality Today: Trends and Controversies.* Sex and Sexuality (vol1); Praeger Publishers; p. 133-152.</u>

15) Palrnore E B. Predictors of the longevity difference: a 25-year follow-up.*Gerontologist*. 1982;6:513-8

16) Westin, L.C. *Can't Orgasm: Here's Help for Women. Originally published in the March/April 2008 issue of* <u>WebMD the Magazine</u>. Retrieved from http://www.webmd.com/sexual-conditions/can't-orgasm-heres-help-for-women

17) Wise, D., Anderson, R. *A Headache in the Pelvis: A new understanding and treatment for prostatitis and chronic pelvic pain syndromes*. 4th ed. National Center for Pelvic Pain Research 2006

Made in the USA
Middletown, DE
04 February 2015